Retreating to Nature

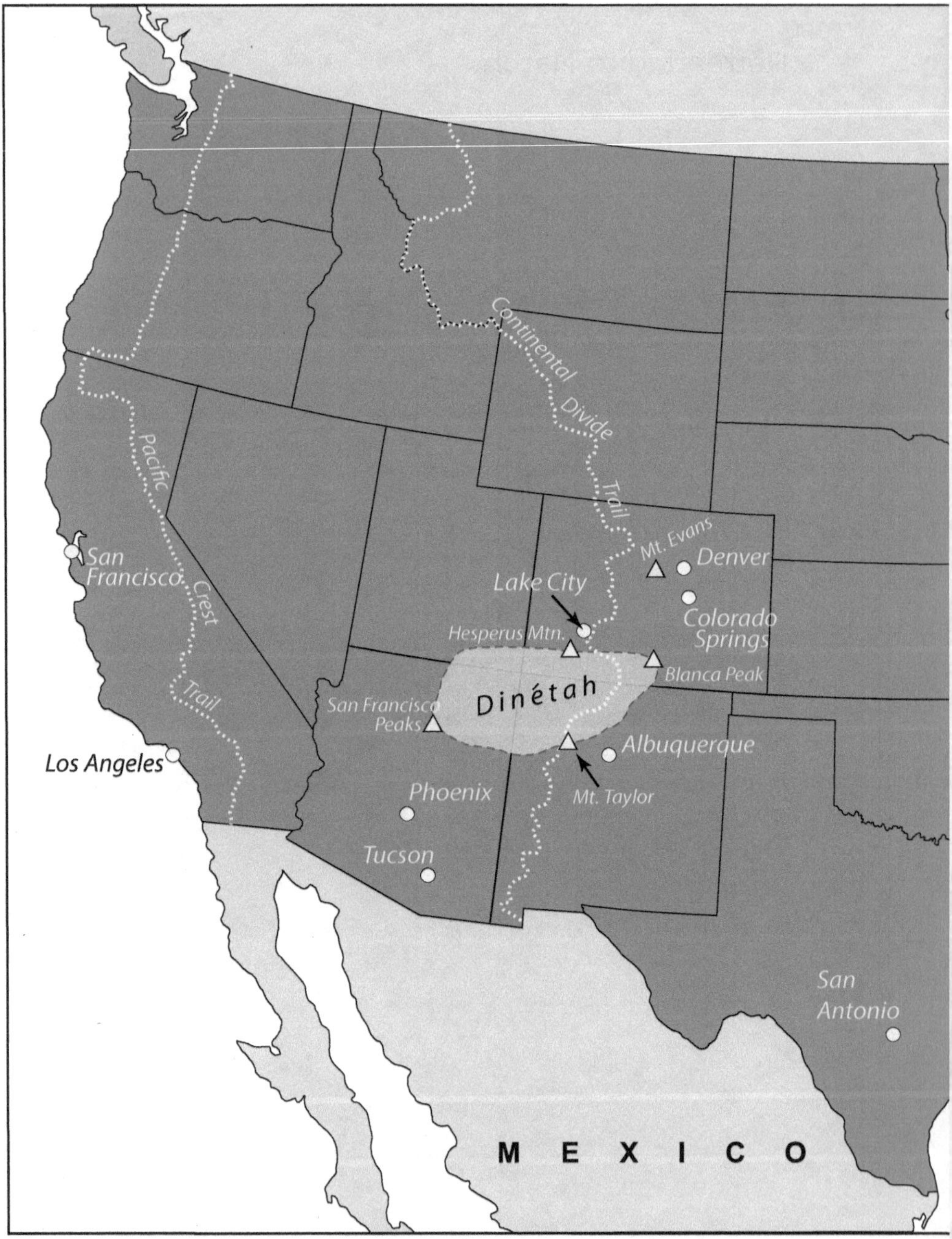

Continental Divide Trail
Pacific Crest Trail
Mt. Evans
Denver
Lake City
Colorado Springs
Hesperus Mtn.
Blanca Peak
Dinétah
San Francisco Peaks
Albuquerque
Mt. Taylor
San Francisco
Los Angeles
Phoenix
Tucson
San Antonio
MEXICO

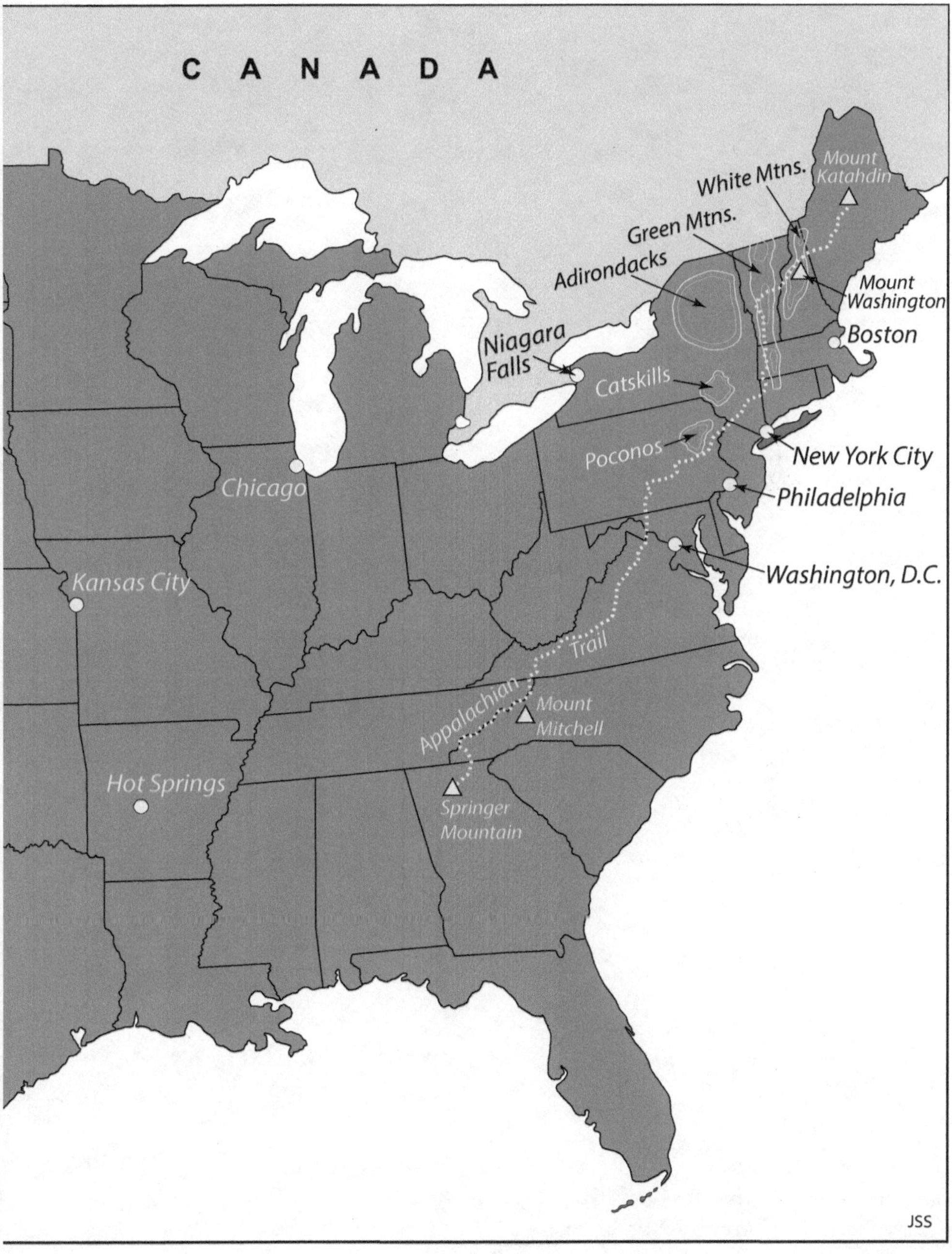

C A N A D A
White Mtns.
Mount Katahdin
Green Mtns.
Adirondacks
Mount Washington
Boston
Niagara Falls
Catskills
Poconos
New York City
Chicago
Philadelphia
Washington, D.C.
Kansas City
Appalachian Trail
Mount Mitchell
Hot Springs
Springer Mountain
JSS

Retreating to Nature

Tracing America's Pursuit of Healing and Restoration

Jeffrey S. Smith

JOHNS HOPKINS UNIVERSITY PRESS BALTIMORE

First printed in the United States of America on acid-free paper
9 8 7 6 5 4 3 2 1

Johns Hopkins University Press
2715 North Charles Street
Baltimore, Maryland 21218
www.press.jhu.edu

Library of Congress Cataloging-in-Publication Data is available.
A catalog record for this book is available from the British Library.

ISBN 978-1-4214-5601-0 (paperback)
ISBN 978-1-4214-5602-7 (ebook)

EU GPSR Authorized Representative
LOGOS EUROPE, 9 rue Nicolas Poussin, 17000, La Rochelle, France
E-mail: Contact@logoseurope.eu

Dedicated to my amazing, wonderful wife, Kim,
who has been at my side through good times and bad.

Your unwavering support has made my
achievements possible.

Thank you for being my best friend!

G.A.D.

Contents

Illustrations

Figures

Tables

Acknowledgments

Writing this book took significant time and effort, but it was also a collaborative endeavor. I deeply appreciate the support and assistance I have received.

First, I extend a heartfelt thank you to the librarians at Kansas State University and the dedicated staff (especially Kathy Coleman) from the Office of Interlibrary Loans, who responded so quickly to my numerous requests. I am also grateful to my department head (Charles Martin) for his unwavering support and encouragement throughout the process. He granted me the latitude and flexibility to engage in a project with a longer-than-average timeline.

I also want to express my gratitude to my friends, colleagues, and relatives who provided invaluable feedback and support throughout the process. Special thanks to Douglas Hurt, Tim Dayton, Geoffrey Buckley, William Wyckoff, Jesus Trevino, Patrick May, Rex "RJ" Rowley, Tim Anderson, Ernesto Vigil, Barney Warf, Sande Williams, Roger Larson, Chris Post, James R. "Pete" Shortridge, Kevin Blake, Audrey Joslin, Paula Bostrom, Ellen Luke, Kathy Zimmerman, Barbara Salazar, Flora and Armando Romero, Maryanne Montoya, and Elizabeth Palizzi. I also thank the students in my various seminars for their thoughtful contributions.

Throughout the process, the editorial team at Johns Hopkins University Press (particularly Robin Coleman) was exceptionally supportive. I am also deeply grateful to the anonymous reviewers for their insightful comments.

My deepest thanks go to my parents (Edwin and Barbara Smith) and my father- and mother-in-law (Paul and Lillian Bostrom). Each of you inspired me and provided a foundation upon which I have built my career. Thank you sincerely.

Note to Reader

This book blends historical narrative, cultural and humanistic geography, and interdisciplinary social-science analysis to trace how Americans have turned to nature-based settings for healing and restoration. Its central focus is the character of "restorative places" across US history, particularly how they emerged, how they have been shaped by social and cultural forces, and why they continue to matter.

To keep the text accessible, technical terminology from geography, environmental psychology, and related fields is used sparingly. Concepts such as therapeutic landscapes, Attention Restoration Theory, and Psycho-Evolutionary Theory are introduced briefly at first mention and revisited only as needed to support the discussion. While the chapters unfold in roughly chronological order, readers interested in particular themes or periods may move among them without losing track of the larger argument.

This work is not intended as an exhaustive history of American attitudes toward nature, nor as a comprehensive survey of all healing landscapes. Instead, it highlights representative episodes, debates, and environments that collectively reveal broader patterns in the ways Americans have sought physical, emotional, and mental renewal in nature.

All maps, photographs, and field observations reflect conditions at the time of research, and because landscapes inevitably evolve, some features described here may have changed. Quotations from archival materials appear as originally written except where minor edits were made for clarity. When interviews are referenced, they were conducted under standard ethical guidelines, and identifying information has been altered when necessary to protect privacy.

Introduction

In 1846, driven by a steadfast belief in Manifest Destiny, the US government laid claim to a vast stretch of land belonging to Mexico, including coastal California. At the time, Yerba Buena was a small, quiet Mexican village with fewer than 400 residents. Two years later, after the Mexican-American War had ended and California was firmly under American control, James Marshall discovered gold at Sutter's Mill, triggering a population boom that would transform the peaceful village. By 1860, San Francisco had grown to 56,000 residents and had developed into a thriving metropolis, bustling with trade and commerce. Like residents in many other fast-growing US cities, San Franciscans faced widespread crime, congestion, noise, and pollution. Seeking an escape from the less desirable qualities of urban living, the city's wealthy turned to Point Lobos as a restorative sanctuary (Figure I.1).

Charles Butler was the first entrepreneur to invest in the northwestern tip of the San Francisco Peninsula. In 1859, Butler purchased 160 acres on Point Lobos, and by 1863 he had opened an establishment of fine dining known as the Cliff House. At the time, few people visited the inn because it was so remote; the trip between San Francisco and Point Lobos required an arduous, six-mile horse ride over seemingly unending sand dunes. However, those intrepid souls who dared to make the three- to four-hour trek were rewarded with peace and solitude combined with spectacular views of the Pacific Ocean.

One year later, with the aim of facilitating travel, Butler teamed up with State Senator James Buckley to build a toll road between the western edge of San Francisco and Point Lobos. The toll road project cost taxpayers

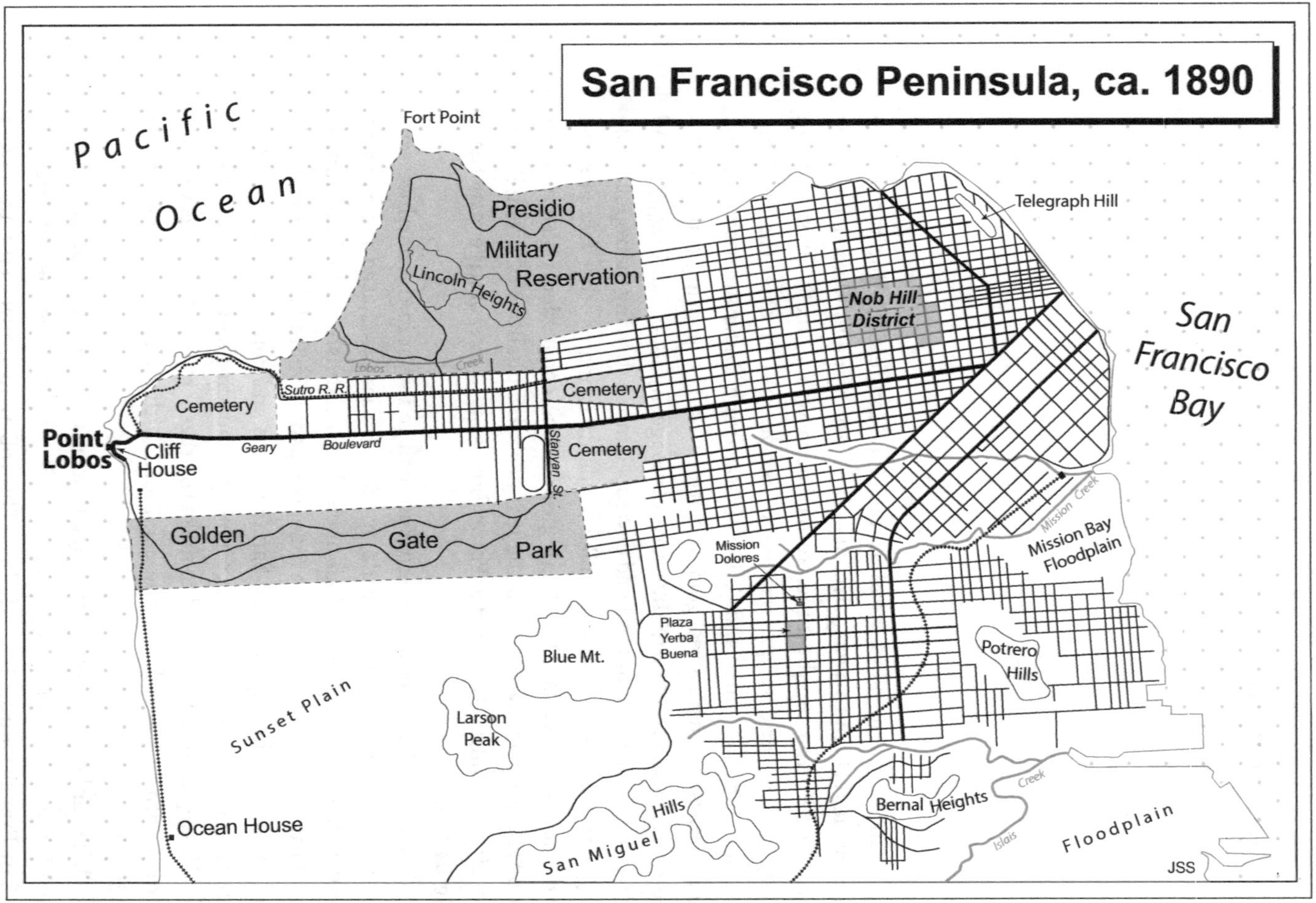

Figure I.1 Map of San Francisco Peninsula, ca. 1890. Cartography by Jeffrey S. Smith.

$175,000 (~$6.7 million today), and cut travel time down to about 30 minutes. At an eye-popping tariff of $1.00 for a round-trip ticket, only the wealthy could afford to use the tollway. The June 25, 1864 issue of the *San Francisco Daily Morning Call* quotes Mark Twain as saying, "If one tires of the drudgeries and scenes of the city, and would breathe the fresh air of the sea, let him take a buggy and pleasant steed, and, ere the sea breeze sets in, glide out to the Cliff House. Away you go over paved roads and make a straight due west course for the ocean. Along the way are many things to please and entertain. The splendid road and ocean air swells the lungs and strengthens the limbs."[1] Cliff House and Point Lobos emerged as a restorative retreat for San Francisco's moneyed elite.

As Cliff House grew in popularity, it became fashionable for the wealthy to embark on a scenic day trip looping from the city to Point Lobos via Fort Point. On their return journey back to their homes in Nob Hill, they passed through an area that would later become Golden Gate Park. On sunny weekends, reports suggest that as many as 1,200 horse-drawn carriages (many bedecked in silver and gold detailing) lined the hitching posts at Cliff House.[2] Butler and his business associates carefully managed all aspects of Cliff House, ensuring a luxurious experience. By the late 1860s, Point Lobos had firmly established itself as the premier scenic retreat for San Francisco's privileged class. However, a dramatic shift in clientele was on the horizon.

Fueled by the wealth generated from gold and silver mining, the City of San Francisco was flush with money. Most of the revenue that flowed into government coffers, however, was used for public construction projects, including schools, roads, piers, and utilities. Despite having ample funds, city planners gave little thought to developing public parks and gardens. When renowned landscape architect Frederick Law Olmsted visited the city, he was struck by the stark contrast between its immense wealth and its lack of public space for rest and recreation. In response, city officials took action in 1871, designating the vast stretch of sand dunes between Stanyan Street and Point Lobos as Golden Gate Park. Six years later, the city completed its first public road through the park, opening the area to a broader segment of the population.

With this new access, middle-class families eagerly ventured to Point Lobos to witness the breathtaking coastal scenery they had long heard about. However, their enthusiasm was short-lived. By the late 1870s, the area had earned a reputation as a playground for young men with money to spare (wealthy heirs and successful miners who indulged in drinking, gambling, and reckless behavior). What had once been a refined, respectable retreat was now notorious for excess and hedonism, driving away the respectable families who had once sought its tranquility.

In March 1881, tycoon Adolph Sutro (a German-born mining engineer and real estate developer) took a carriage ride around Fort Point and south to Ocean Beach. Upon reaching Point Lobos, Sutro became captivated by a small cottage overlooking Cliff House and the Pacific Ocean. Over the next three years, Sutro not only acquired the cottage, but also purchased more than 80 acres of land along this stretch of the Pacific Coast. When he learned about Cliff House's unsavory reputation, his disdain for such debauchery motivated him to buy the establishment. Under the supervision of a newly appointed manager, Sutro restored Cliff House to a respectable venue, one featuring quality dining and family-friendly entertainment. With this transformation underway, Sutro began developing what he called San Francisco's "Outside Lands."

Over the next decade, Sutro completely reshaped the landscape around Point Lobos (Figure I.2). At Cliff House, he expanded the structure, adding a sprawling porch and a glass-paned conservatory that offered spectacular, breathtaking views of the shoreline. In 1883, he began developing his masterpiece, Sutro Heights. The 21-acre property perched on a bluff overlooking Seal Rocks was the ideal location for a parapet observation platform surrounded by lush gardens and a network of hiking trails. According to a 1973 National Park Service report, the original design of Sutro Heights reflects, in part, a deep commitment to preserving the site's remarkable setting and extraordinary natural beauty.[3] Winding pedestrian paths crisscrossed the meticulously manicured gardens, leading visitors from one lookout or seating area to another. To shield the area from harsh coastal winds and prevent soil erosion, workers erected tall wooden fences and planted an assortment of trees. In the process, they also created individual, outdoor garden rooms. These private and secluded outdoor spaces provided visitors with a quiet refuge to connect with nature and take in the soothing, panoramic views of the coastline.

When Sutro Heights opened to the public in 1885, it was an instant success. The Outside Lands became known as "Lands End," a beloved destination where people could gaze out over the ocean or immerse themselves in the serenity of the gardens. Offering a restorative experience for people of all backgrounds, Sutro Heights provided an escape from the harsher

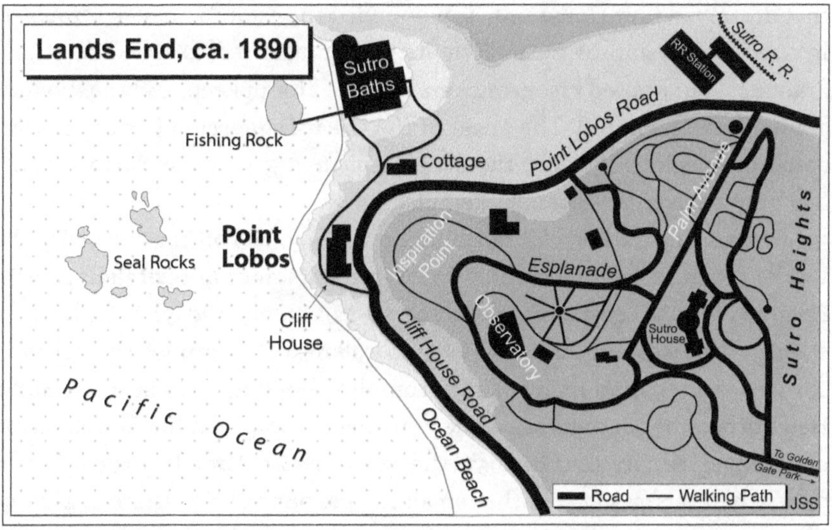

Figure I.2 Map of Lands End, ca. 1890. Cartography by Jeffrey S. Smith.

realities of urban life, a place where individuals could find solace in nature's embrace.

Building upon his passion for natural history and his love for nature, Sutro's next endeavor was the construction of an aquarium. The project began in early 1887 when he successfully petitioned the federal government to designate the habitat around Seal Rocks as a nature preserve. Later that year, the aquarium opened with considerable fanfare, but it was merely the first step in a grander vision Sutro had for the oceanfront property. In 1889, construction began on Sutro's Baths. When the massive, glass-enclosed pavilion was completed in 1896, it featured seven pools (six saltwater and one freshwater) each heated at a different temperature. Designed to accommodate up to 5,500 visitors, Sutro Baths became the world's largest public bathhouse at the time.[4] A visit to Sutro Baths crowned an all-day family excursion to the shore, which often included stops at Ocean Beach, Cliff House, and Sutro Heights.

Following Adolph Sutro's death in 1898, his daughter Emma was left with mounting debts and a failing business plan that was hemorrhaging money. Despite her efforts to maintain the properties, the Sutro Estate (Cliff House, Sutro Baths, and Sutro Heights) fell into decline. A devastating fire in 1907 that destroyed Cliff House only compounded the estate's financial troubles. In 1920, ownership of Sutro Heights was transferred to the City of San Francisco, but limited resources were allocated for upkeep, and the grounds gradually deteriorated. The onset of the Great Depression further exacerbated the neglect. By 1935, the once-manicured gardens at Sutro Heights had become overgrown and unkempt.

Recognizing the need for rehabilitation, in 1937 city officials turned to the Works Progress Administration (WPA) for assistance in revitalizing Sutro Heights Park. At a cost of nearly $91,000 (~$2.1 million today), WPA workers stabilized the western cliffs, widened the walking paths, pruned the trees and shrubs, and repaired many of the crumbling buildings. Once again, Sutro Heights became a haven for people yearning to escape the hustle and bustle of a congested city life. In 1951, the Sutro era at Point Lobos came to a close when the family sold the remaining portions of the estate to George Whitney. The new owner steered the business in a decidedly different direction, away from its original emphasis on nature, signaling the close of a remarkable chapter in San Francisco's history.

Since the mid-1850s, Point Lobos and the Sutro Historic District have been used by San Francisco residents as a place of diversion from everyday routines and an escape from the stresses and strains of urban living. Most historical accounts of Lands End focus on the evolving array of dining, entertainment, and leisure opportunities that the oceanfront businesses (especially Cliff House) have offered. Such accounts, however, downplay the fact that the foundation of Lands End has always been its magnificent natural setting and scenic beauty. During its heyday in the 1890s, Point Lobos offered a wide variety of nature-based attractions, including beachcombing and sunbathing at Ocean Beach, relishing the spectacular views of Seal Rocks from Cliff House, soaking and swimming at Sutro Baths, walking through the peaceful gardens at Sutro Heights, and engaging in leisure activities at Golden Gate Park. From panoramic views of the coastline and observing endemic plant and animal communities to walking, hiking, and bathing, the northwest coast of the San Francisco Peninsula has always been a place where city dwellers could retreat to nature and find personal restoration.

The foregoing narrative of Lands End serves as a compelling illustration of this book's central purpose. Its aim is to examine pivotal milestones and select sociocultural forces in US history that have shaped how nature-based places have been used as a tool to combat mental, emotional, and physical disease. Nature has long been used as a resource for convalescence because it enables people to distance themselves from the hectic aspects of their lives and affords individuals space to rest, recharge, and recover both mentally and physically. Residents of San Francisco have not only shared Adolph Sutro's love of nature, but they have availed themselves of nature's healing and restorative qualities found at Lands End.

As many of the examples and case studies presented in this book reveal, it was typically the wealthy who led the charge to nature because they had the time and financial resources to explore remote lands. Point Lobos was no different. In the early years, affluent families from San Francisco, as well as a host of celebrities and dignitaries (including Presidents Grant, Hayes, McKinley, Roosevelt, and Taft), ventured to the margins of the San Francisco Peninsula to enjoy the peaceful, breathtaking views and spend time soaking up the life-giving qualities of nature. As transportation technology improved and new labor laws awarded wage-earning individuals more leisure time, households of modest means began following in the footsteps of the wealthy. Middle-class families then had the opportunity to escape the stresses of urban living and embrace the recharging, restorative qualities of nature. The various accounts presented in this book also speak to the guiding force of innovative entrepreneurs and visionary professionals, as well as the role of local governments in establishing parks and other nature-based places for personal restoration.

Lands End is one of an untold number of places across the country that continues to benefit from the foresight of leading local citizens. As will be presented throughout the subsequent chapters, their endeavors are still paying dividends today. The focus of this book is to illuminate the historic foundations and geographic contexts that gave rise to modern, nature-based restorative places. To better understand nature's role in treating mental and physical ailments today, it is helpful to look to the past for insights.

History of Alleviating Mental and Physical Disease

As early as 2,500 BC, the ancient Babylonians, Egyptians, and Chinese were among the earliest to explore remedies for depression and other mental health issues. They believed that poor mental health resulted from demons or evil spirits overcoming a person's body. Pagan religious leaders would treat the afflicted individual with prayer and exorcisms, including beatings, physical restraint, and starvation.[5] Two millennia later, wisdom among ancient Greeks was divided; some still espousing the evil spirit origins, while others advanced a more modern perspective centered on an individual's overall mental and physical health.

The earliest account to consider melancholia and sadness as a mental health disorder was recorded in the tenth century by a Persian physician (Abu Ali Husain Ibn Sina, better known as Avicenna) who treated depression with various herbs, music therapy, and positive reinforcement.[6] By the early 1800s, depression was largely regarded as a mental weakness in an individual's battle between good and bad, right and wrong. Experts at the time called for treatments, including dietary changes, electric shock, enemas, and water immersion. Some even believed that a rigorous horseback ride would jar the brain back into its correct position.[7]

Aside from treating common blunt force injuries like abrasions, contusions, fractures, and lacerations that have long plagued humanity, early medical professionals were also dedicated to alleviating diseases linked to poor mental health and addressing a diverse array of physical ailments. One enduring example is the practice of soaking in geothermal waters, a remedy that has been practiced for thousands of years. First introduced by the Aegeans, warm water therapy was known to relieve muscle tension, ease joint pain, and cure skin conditions. Throughout history, numerous other nature-based therapies have been introduced and later abandoned, such as the use of leeches and maggots, bloodletting, and even consuming skunk soup to treat colds. While each aimed to relieve illness and physical discomfort, their effectiveness varied significantly.

Today, there are a slew of modern treatment options for poor mental health including an alphabet soup of pharmaceutical therapies (SSRIs, SNRIs, tricyclic and tetracyclic antidepressants, MAOIs, NMDAs) as well as everything from aromatherapy to yoga. An exhaustive examination of the various treatments to combat mental health disorders is well beyond the scope of this book. Suffice it to say that in addition to professional counseling and prescription medications, an entire self-help industry has sprung up to assist individuals overcome mental health disorders. In fact, some of the most aggressive marketing schemes over the past decade (e.g., gravity blankets, adult coloring books, fidget toys) were designed to promote happiness and contentment.

In his book, *The Depression Cure*, psychologist Stephen Ilardi recommends the use of natural remedies (e.g., healthy eating, positive thinking, physical exercise, restorative sleep) to combat poor mental health and physical disease.[8] Central to his advice is spending time in nature, a practice substantiated by a growing body of research that asserts our minds are inherently drawn to the outdoors because having contact with nature improves mental health.[9] Supporting this idea, researchers George MacKerron and Susana Mourato analyzed crowdsourced data from 20,000 participants worldwide to explore the connection between environmental conditions and feelings of happiness and favorable mental health. Their findings reveal that individuals across all demographic groups are significantly happier in nature-based settings compared to urban environments.[10]

Although there is a considerable and growing body of research that speaks to the known health benefits of spending time in nature, there is little scholarship that explores the history of restorative places. What lessons from history can be found to enhance our understanding of nature's role in easing mental and physical distress? The purpose of this book is to examine pivotal milestones and select sociocultural forces in US history that shaped how nature-based places have been used as a tool to combat mental, emotional, and physical disease. The focus is on understanding the historic and geographic contexts that gave rise to modern restorative places.

Defining Restorative Places

In her review of existing literature, Rita Berto suggests that restorative places are settings that facilitate the renewal of personal adaptive resources.[11] In essence, these locations help neutralize the stresses of modern urban living, aid in quieting the mind, enable physical convalescence, nurture a healthy spirit, promote emotional tranquility, and restore mental capacity. Ultimately, restorative places help reduce mental fatigue and restore an individual's ability to cope with the sensory overload often linked to urban environments.

Upon closer inspection, restorative places have two main aspects. First, they are places that offer an escape from the stresses of life's daily routines. As such, most restorative places are a wellspring of peace, harmony, serenity, and solitude. These soothing environments tend to be welcoming, comforting, calming, and empowering. This perspective focuses on the ambient qualities of restorative places. Second, restorative places are environments that promote healing and improve an individual's mental and physical well-being. They are nurturing places where renewal, recovery, and strengthening unfold. When combined, both the calming and curative qualities of restorative places improve levels of personal satisfaction and allow for self-realization.[12]

Restorative places are as individualistic as people themselves; they vary by age, ancestry, culture, gender, and income. Moreover, restorative environments can be both natural and man-made. For example, research suggests that some people feel recharged and rejuvenated after going to a shopping mall, gambling casino, or fitness center.[13] Such individuals thrive on excitement and adrenaline rushes where abundant amounts of dopamine are released into their endocrine system. Others find peace and comfort in quiet locations. Relatively new research reveals that the quietude of libraries, museums, and art galleries is stress relieving and restorative.[14] It bears repeating that what is inspirational and invigorating to one person may not be to another. Despite the great diversity in places, a sizable body of literature concludes that the restoration process is most effective in natural settings with abundant vegetation and beautiful scenery.[15]

As illustrated throughout this book, restorative places also transcend time and culture. Throughout history, Indigenous Peoples have identified places as sacred because they embody the symbiotic relationship between all living things and foster a connection between the living world and the spirit world. Such places have aided First Peoples in communing with nature and enabled them to engage in activities that promote a healthy spirit and rejuvenate the mind, body, and soul. Today, people of all backgrounds draw similar inspiration from many of the same places because they promote physical convalescence, emotional healing, and spiritual renewal.

A compelling example can be found in the *Diné* (Navajo) culture, which recognizes four sacred peaks demarcating the boundaries of *Dinétah* (the Navajo Homeland) (Figure I.3). To the *Diné*, the four mountains represent the dwelling places of deities who safeguard vital resources and embody supernatural power. Through specific rituals, the Navajo can access and release the power held within each peak. As Stephen Jett explains, "most of the ceremonies [associated with the four sacred peaks] relate directly to the restoration, maintenance or acquisition of health, harmony, and well-being."[16]

Of particular significance is Tsoodził (also known as Mount Taylor), located near Grants, New Mexico. According to *Diné* legend, First Man

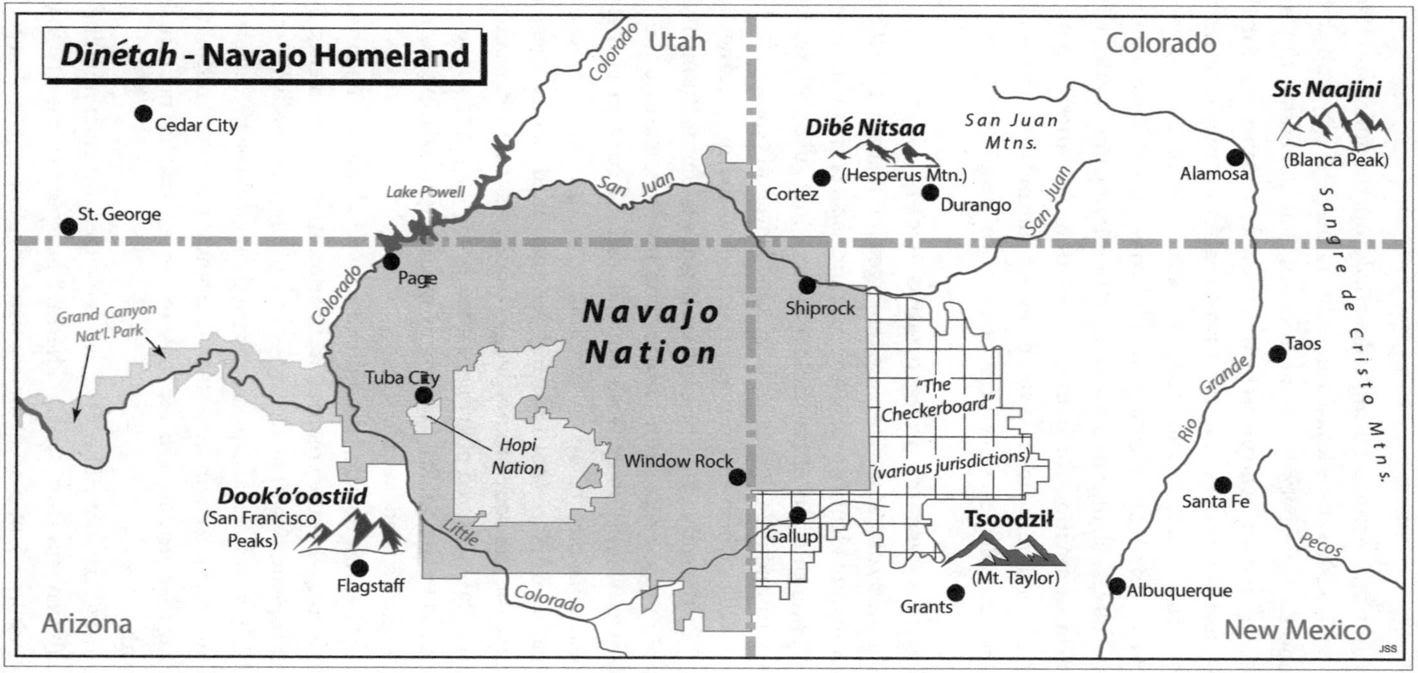

Figure I.3 Map of *Dinétah*. Cartography by Jeffrey S. Smith.

shaped Turquoise Mountain using soil carried from the underworld, securing it to the earth with a stone knife. Not only did the peak play a pivotal role in the cosmic struggle between good and evil, but it became the home of Turquoise Boy and Girl, who protect the precious blue stones found in the area. Tsoodził remains a sacred site where Navajo healers and religious practitioners gather feathers, pollen, soil, and turquoise stones for restorative ceremonies such as the *Hózhóóji* (The Blessing Way).[17] Today, Mount Taylor continues to hold deep cultural significance for Native American communities while also serving as a destination for outdoor recreation. Activities such as hiking, camping, and endurance racing extend beyond cultural boundaries, offering a mental and psychological retreat for thousands of people each year.

Existing Research on Restorative Places

The study of restorative places emerged indirectly in the late 1950s as scholars sought to identify urban stressors and aspects of environmental aesthetics. During this period, psychologists were intrigued with understanding the environmental triggers for heightened levels of stress and emotional arousal, as well as which environments people find soothing and aesthetically pleasing.[18] By the early 1970s, researchers began examining the mental health benefits of outdoor recreation. During the 1990s, research on restorative places surged when Wilbert Gesler introduced the concept of therapeutic landscapes. With a focus on understanding the intersection between the characteristics of place (both natural and man-made landscapes) and the healing process, the body of knowledge steadily moved from examining extraordinary places (sacred pilgrimage sites, hot springs and spa towns, spiritual retreats) to the qualities of everyday settings (coastlines, community gardens, libraries, woodlands).[19]

During the same decade, environmental psychologists joined the fray and began exploring what they referred to as restorative environments. Scholars, mainly European, began aggressively examining the ambient conditions under which an individual experiences psychological resource depletion (i.e., stressed out) and the environments that promote emotional restoration. Two overlapping theories emerged and most of the research has fallen in line with one or both.

Psycho-Evolutionary Theory (PET) is focused on understanding how an individual recovers from stress. The PET perspective asserts that stress recovery occurs when a scene or ambient environment evokes feelings of interest, pleasantness, and tranquility. The process unfolds in the following manner: a scene or environment with sufficient complexity and natural content (vegetation, water) elicits interest and positive affect, thereby displacing or mitigating negative thoughts, and allows for autonomic arousal to drop to more moderate levels.[20] Restoration results in lower blood pressure, reduced muscle tension, and an increase in positive emotions.

The other favored psychological perspective is Attention Restoration Theory (ART) which is concerned with restoration from attention fatigue. According to ART, it is assumed that, by default, individuals are not interested in or focused on the task(s) at hand; the brain would much rather be doing something else. Thus, the individual must employ a central inhibitory capacity (mechanism) that will inhibit competing thoughts or stimuli. Over time, the effort it takes to achieve focus leads to mental fatigue and emotional stress. The individual becomes irritable, fails to recognize interpersonal cues, loses self-control, and the quality of their work suffers.[21] To counteract the diminished capacity to concentrate, the person must experience fascination. Fascination is any involuntary activity (does not require mental or emotional energy) that allows an individual to gain psychological distance from the task(s) at hand (i.e., check out). Natural environments are deemed most effective in enabling an individual to "get away" because there is an absence of daily stressors and there are sufficient aesthetically pleasing features such as natural light, vegetation, water, and animals that evoke fascination.[22]

Building on the foundation established by these two dominant theories, and utilizing highly quantitative methods, environmental psychologists are rapidly advancing the field. Scholars continue to broaden the scope of understanding by examining how diverse outdoor spaces and indoor settings (e.g., houses of worship, museums, art galleries) function as restorative environments.[23] Simultaneously, other researchers are delving deeper into the specific mechanisms underlying the restorative process. Their work explores various antecedent conditions that contribute to heightened stress levels,[24] the varying environmental characteristics of restorative places,[25] and the distinctions between actual and perceived outcomes associated with restorative experiences.[26]

The ongoing pursuit to better understand restorative environments has led scholars to develop indices measuring the restorativeness of different places.[27] Among the most significant contributions is the work of Terry Hartig and his colleagues, who have identified four key factors that form the basis of the Perceived Restorativeness Scale (PRS).[28] Testing a variety of variables and environmental conditions, their index asserts that the restorative process is most effective in places where individuals can distance themselves from life's stressors (being away). In this first factor, physical and mental detachment from stressful environments is vital, but the quality of the restorative experience is also important. Thus, the second factor (extent) refers to how well an individual relates to and perceives the restorative environment. In other words, is the place a good fit with an individual's personal preferences, and how do individuals perceive the restorative environment? Restoration is most effective when people develop an emotional attachment to the place and there are abundant opportunities for mental diversion.[29] Existing research concludes that extent can be experienced through immersion in actual physical environments as well as intellectual activities (such as viewing photos, videos, and virtual reality).[30] Fascination, the third factor, relates to the conditions which enable an individual to release their mind from active engagement. The simple act of walking in the woods, painting by numbers, or daydreaming requires little cognitive energy, thus allowing the brain to rejuvenate and restore its capacity to function properly. Finally, compatibility refers to the match between a person's goals or intentions and the demands made on the individual by environmental conditions. The restoration process is most successful when there is a high level of compatibility between what a person wants to achieve and the environment's suitability in meeting that goal. Although extensive research has examined specific environmental variables that promote restoration and identified which settings best support individual healing, relatively little attention has been given to the major milestones or sociocultural forces in US history that shaped how nature has been used as a tool to promote personal restoration.

The research conducted by environmental psychologists is closely linked with ongoing work in architecture and landscape design. Designers have long recognized that the integration of buildings and natural elements creates spaces that are both aesthetically pleasing and conducive to personal well-being. As William Browning and Catherine Ryan write, "when people are regularly in contact with nature, personal health and well-being will improve in a manner and to a degree that contributes to public health, community resilience and environmental stewardship."[31] In essence, individuals experience greater happiness and improved mental and physical health when the built environment they occupy incorporates both direct and indirect connections to nature.

Over the course of his seventy-year career, a majority of Frank Lloyd Wright's architectural designs embody this concept. As founder of the organic-architecture movement, he advocated for harmony between the built environment and nature. His structures contain strong horizontal elements that emphasize connections to the ground and liberal use of glass that breaks down the barrier between inside and outside spaces. This is best exemplified in his design of Fallingwater (completed in 1939), where the layout and positioning of the private dwelling meld with the natural setting.

The inspiration for this book came from a volume edited by William Wyckoff and Lary Dilsaver, which traces the sequent occupance of the mountainous West. Their anthology identifies five geographic themes that define the distinctive American subregion, including a section dedicated to the restorative qualities of mountains. As they explain, the idea of mountains as restorative sanctuaries "is an outgrowth of late nineteenth-century Romanticism, which envisaged many western mountain settings as healthy and idyllic retreats from the increasingly urbanized and fast-paced world beyond."[32] Although this book shares Wyckoff and Dilsaver's foundation in cultural-historical geography, it takes a distinctly humanistic approach.

As a cognate field to environmental psychology, landscape architecture, and environmental history, humanistic geography seeks to understand people's relationship with places and geographical environments.[33] At its core, the humanistic approach is driven to understand and articulate a sense of place over time. Popularized by John Brinckerhoff (J. B.) Jackson, sense of place is a complex construct that encompasses both the distinctive qualities and characteristics of a location, as well as the physical, intellectual, and emotional experiences people associate with that place.[34]

The concept of sense of place is closely tied to phenomenology, which frames the study of place as a meaningful location created through human experience. The strength of the phenomenological perspective is its focus on exposing the taken-for-granted experiences of everyday geographic phenomena such as home, work, and play.[35] Thus, this book advances scholarship that seeks to understand how meaningful places are created by human activity, as well as how places shape future human action and experience.

In 1992, Wilbert Gesler coined the phrase "therapeutic landscapes" to describe a new subfield within cultural geography that seeks to identify physical, cultural, and symbolic landscapes (environments) that are associated with favorable health. As Gesler explains, these settings can include traditional (e.g., brick-and-mortar) landscapes like health spas and monastery retreats, as well as nontraditional (e.g., intangible) landscapes, such as representations of place in art and literature.[36] In her thorough review of the subfield, Allison Williams explains that research on therapeutic landscapes can be distilled to three substantive areas. First are physical places reputed for health and healing such as care facilities and wellness spas. Second is the transformation or shift of healthcare sites from a treatment-oriented approach to one centered on prevention. Gardens and substance abuse recovery centers fall under this category. Third are spaces that are significant to a particular population such as pilgrimage and sacred sites. In all cases, therapeutic landscapes have an enduring reputation for achieving physical, mental, and spiritual healing.[37]

Although there is a broad body of work on restorative places, including contributions from environmental psychologists, landscape architects, and cultural geographers, few studies have explored restorative places from a historical perspective. Specifically, there is a lack of research that seeks to understand the larger sociocultural forces that gave rise to the idea that natural settings provide significant restorative benefits (physically, mentally, and emotionally). This book helps fill that gap in the literature by exploring how restorative places that center on nature have been a recurring theme in American history. The purpose of this book is to examine pivotal milestones and select sociocultural forces in US history that shaped how nature-based places have been used as a tool to promote personal restoration. The book's content addresses such questions as, what were the inspirational beginnings of restorative places, what places first served as retreats from the unseemly elements of modern urban living, what institutional and technological changes in society precipitated the rise of restorative places for the masses, where have urban-dwelling residents found refuge within their own cities, and how has nature been used as a restorative tool in the healing process throughout history? Although the book's focus is on understanding major milestones in US history, some chapters present events and conditions outside North America because they provide relevant background and historical context for what has unfolded within the United States.

Organization of the Book

This introductory chapter provides historical background on addressing mental and physical disease, defines restorative places, summarizes seminal research, and highlights the synergy between disciplinary approaches. The remainder of this book is divided into five content chapters and a conclusion. Chapter 1 explores the early nineteenth-century debate over America's trajectory. On one side, government officials and business leaders pushed for land development, viewing nature as an obstacle to progress that needed to be conquered. On the other, a renowned group of scholars, philosophers, and writers challenged the prevailing mindset, expressing grave concerns about the senseless destruction of wilderness. As the Transcendentalist movement's leading spokesperson, Henry David Thoreau railed against the dehumanizing aspects of industrialization and advocated for regarding nature as a remedy for the damaged human condition and a source of personal restoration. The chapter then shows that transcendentalism inspired America's first homegrown art movement, gave form and substance to transcendentalist ideas, and further shaped how the public thought about the natural environment. Scholars have bifurcated the artists of the Hudson River School of landscape painting, but the commonality among both generations was their awe-inspiring depiction of nature's majestic qualities, attention to detail, and their determination to capture a view of nature that would afford people a respite from the stressors of everyday life.

The next two chapters work in tandem to examine the emergence of places offering refuge from the excesses of urban living. Chapter 2 highlights destinations popular among America's upper crust. It begins with mountainous retreats in the Pocono and Catskill Mountains and then digs into the growing popularity of the Adirondacks. In succession, the wealthy rented cabins, stayed in opulent resorts, and built summer retreats (great camps) in these mountainous regions. As the middle class began discovering the natural beauty of the eastern uplands, the rich began colonizing the White Mountains of New Hampshire. Time spent surrounded by nature provided them with cool mountain air, rest in peaceful tranquility, and the opportunity to recharge their mental and physical capacities. Of note is the opening of Crawford Path. Not only did the nation's oldest continuously used hiking trail inspire urban elite to form hiking and adventure clubs, but it served as a catalyst for developing the Appalachian Trail. Highlighting the creation of the Appalachian Trail with its inherent restorative qualities serves as a robust transition to the next chapter, which focuses on key sociocultural events in US history that enabled America's masses to enjoy nature's restorative qualities.

During the nearly four decades spanning the Gilded Age and the Progressive Era, America made an untold number of remarkable transformations, none more significant to the concept of restorative places than labor reform. The nation shifted from one dominated by ruthless business transactions, uninhibited greed, and worker exploitation to one that rebuked big business, valued environmental conservation, and championed labor rights. Chapter 3 traces how the labor reform movement and rise of mass-produced automobiles gave the working class greater access to nature. After decades of lockouts and labor strikes, the establishment of a 40-hour workweek provided workers with both sufficient income and ample leisure time. Moreover, the private automobiles afforded middle-class Americans the wherewithal to travel at their own pace and choose their own destinations. Sunday drives in the country became a balm for the worn-out city soul. Many cities leveraged the car culture's economic potential, but Denver, Colorado, led the nation in creating the first mountain park system. In 1912, city officials approved a plan to build looping roads into the nearby mountains, giving residents of the Mile High City access to clean air, cooler temperatures, and invigorating natural settings. The chapter highlights several noteworthy locations, including Red Rocks Amphitheater, Mount Evans, and the Lariat Loop. These mountain footholds were designed not only to offer scenic drives for those with newly acquired automobiles and encourage new business ventures, but also to create spaces where people could relax, recharge, and reconnect with nature. In 1972, as Denver's Mountain Parks were falling into disrepair, neighboring Jefferson County established its own Open Space program to preserve natural areas. With the goal of improving community health, city governments throughout the Denver metropolitan area have continued to safeguard open space as a place where people can find restoration.

As people came to recognize the restorative qualities of nature that lie beyond city limits, visionary leaders sought to introduce those same benefits into the urban fabric. William Cullen Bryant, for example, was a staunch advocate for city parks and ardently believed that individuals overwhelmed by the "sorrows, crimes, and incivility of cities" should have the chance to "enter the woods and view the haunts of nature" to experience peace and serenity.[38] Chapter 4 traces the historical progression of how city officials have set aside space within cities for personal restoration. It begins by considering the remarkable work of Frederick Law Olmsted, whose vision for Central Park not only created a restorative place within New York City, but laid the groundwork for the City Beautiful Movement. The chapter then examines Chicago's World's Fair and Washington DC's National Mall as examples of how a city could be both functional and restorative. Over subsequent decades, many midsized cities, like Birmingham, Buffalo, and Milwaukee, followed their lead. With its abundant tree-lined boulevards, bubbling fountains, scenic parkways, and public parks, no city has done more to embrace the City Beautiful Movement than Kansas City, Missouri. Those investments are still paying dividends today.

At times, certain places become recognized as restorative because their distinctive natural features are believed to promote well-being. Chapter 5 examines two compelling examples of therapeutic destinations in the United States that rose to prominence due to the perception that their inherent characteristics foster healing, renewal, and personal restoration. In 1832, the US government designated Hot Springs, Arkansas, as a Federal Reservation, and fifty years later it established the country's first health spa. By the turn of the century, people suffering from a variety of physical ailments found their way to the Ouachita Mountains of west-central Arkansas. Initially a destination for treating physical maladies, the area evolved into a restorative place that treated people holistically (the mind as well as the body). Key to the healing process was a network of color-coded hiking trails, which allowed visitors to experience the serenity of the nearby forested mountains after soaking in one of the area's warm mineral bathhouses. Around the same time, tuberculosis was a raging infirmity that plagued society. Doctors often prescribed a trip to the thin, dry air of the American West for people afflicted with pulmonary consumption. Albuquerque, Denver, Phoenix, Tucson, San Antonio, and San Diego saw their populations grow from the influx of "lungers" seeking relief. Although many cities in the West became restorative places for people suffering from the debilitating malady, Colorado Springs received a disproportionate share of patients. Because investors opened so many sanatoria at the base of Pikes Peak, for about fifty years the town's identity was largely shaped by tuberculosis.[39] As antibiotics revolutionized medicine, the need for health spas and convalescent centers declined. Most closed or were converted into other uses.

Today, approximately 1.2 billion people worldwide (about 15 percent of the global population) suffer from a continuum of mental health disorders. In the US, 19 percent of adults experience some form of mental illness each year.[40] Sensory overload and overcrowding are the two biggest challenges associated with urban living, making access to restorative places essential. Individuals find renewal and restoration in countless ways, but it is effectively achieved when people have a place where they can retreat (escape) from the physical, mental, and emotional stressors of city life. Research indicates that interacting with nature is an optimal way to improve mental, physical, and spiritual health. This book's central aim is to examine pivotal milestones and select sociocultural forces in US history that have shaped how nature-based places have been used as a tool to combat mental, emotional, and physical disease. Rather than following a purely chronological order, this book uses historical case studies to highlight the foundations and geographic contexts that gave rise to modern, nature-based restorative places. By examining the past, the book offers insights into nature's role in contemporary health and wellness. The concluding chapter synthesizes common themes from the five preceding chapters and reinforces our current understanding of restorative places. Finally, because this book is rooted in humanistic geography, it also examines the emotional connections people form with everyday spaces, deepening our appreciation of place and its role in fostering well-being.

1

Roots of Restoration

Transcendentalism and the Hudson River School of Landscape Painting

In the years following the American Revolutionary War, the fledgling nation was marked by overwhelming confidence and euphoria. Having thrown off the shackles of British imperialism, America was primed for growth and achievement. Furthermore, as the Industrial Revolution took hold, remarkable scientific inventions were ushering in astounding changes within society. Over the course of a few short decades households acquired reliable radiant heat, indoor plumbing, and incandescent lighting. Optimism prevailed because the quality of life for many families seemed to be improving.

In the midst of the country's remarkable achievements, however, there was a groundswell of discontent. Scholars, philosophers, theologians, and writers witnessed another side of American society that was rife with urban overcrowding, inadequate housing, lack of public transportation, air and water pollution, rampant crime, and interpersonal conflict. Moreover, industrial magnates were exploiting people of all races and backgrounds in their pursuit of financial gain. The leading thinkers of the day proclaimed that American society's gyroscope was off kilter; the country had lost its moral compass.

On September 8, 1836, a group of New England-based luminaries, inspired by the works of philosophers Emanuel Swedenborg and Immanuel Kant, gathered at Willard's Hotel in Cambridge, Massachusetts, to discuss the unsatisfactory state of affairs within American society (Richardson 1995). The informal gatherings became known as the symposium of the Transcendental Club. Members of the club engaged in civic debate and drew attention to the ills of society. Between 1840 and 1929, the club published an array of articles addressing a number of social issues, particularly women's rights, universal human equality, and the fair treatment of laborers.

The Transcendentalist Movement, closely associated with American Romanticism, was a reaction to modernist thinking. Transcendentalism harkened back to Thomas Jefferson's notions of the ideal society. Having condemned cities as centers of vice and hedonism, Jefferson adamantly asserted that yeoman farmers (simple folk who work the land) are God's chosen people because they live clean lives and embody the virtues of humanity.[1] By the mid-nineteenth century, transcendentalism had evolved into a complex, multifaceted perspective on life that is difficult to pin down. At its core, the movement encouraged people to be self-reliant, live a simple life free of external influences, and above all relish in the beauty (divinity) of nature. Particularly relevant to this book is that the transcendentalists praised efforts to get back to nature in whatever form it takes (gardening, hiking, traveling, painting) because such actions provide an escape from the frantic pace of increasing industrialization, the stresses of everyday urban living, and growing social conflict. The list of notable transcendentalists is considerably long including academics, artists, journalists, ministers, poets, and politicians. None, however, were more influential than Ralph Waldo Emerson and Henry David Thoreau.

As an ardent critic of modern industrial society, Emerson prevailed upon American citizens to abandon modern ways of life fraught with distractions and material obsessions. Instead, he encouraged them to cultivate self-reliance, cherish individual freedoms, embrace the simple beauty of daily existence, and develop a harmonious connection with nature. Over the course of his career, the father of the Transcendentalist Movement published hundreds of books and essays and delivered thousands of public lectures. In his most influential publication (*Nature*), Emerson articulates the core element of transcendentalism; with all its beauty, nature is at the center of life. In the book he asserts that instead of chasing a fleeting, ever-elusive form of happiness based on modern, urban living, people should slow down, embrace nature, and immerse themselves in the childlike innocence and life-giving aspects of the woods, meadows, and streams. For example, he writes: "In the woods, is perpetual youth. . . . In the woods, we return to reason and faith. There I feel that nothing can befall me in life, no disgrace, no calamity, which nature cannot repair."[2]

Overall, Emerson's writings align with both major theories concerning restorative places. He advanced the notion that nature offers profound interest and tranquility, reflecting the core principles of Psycho-Evolutionary Theory. Likewise, in keeping with the tenets of Attention Restoration Theory, Emerson regarded nature as inherently beautiful, capable of inspiring fascination and granting individuals the mental space needed to distance themselves from stress.

Given the prominent role he held among the transcendentalists, Emerson undoubtedly helped shape the thinking of his contemporaries. Throughout his career, Emerson saw the unfolding beauty of nature as artwork; each dewdrop, each flower petal, each leaf is the artistic expression of the divine. In his mind, however, few adults can see nature in that manner. Instead, it takes a trained eye to discern the true beauty of nature in all its seasons.

In August 1858, Emerson and nine other members of Boston's Saturday Club participated in a two-week camping trip to the Adirondack Mountains in upstate New York. The group of philosophers and politicians, authors and artists, and other like-minded intellectuals spent their days exploring the wonders of the woods and their nights debating the virtues of nature. The adventure at Follensby Pond had a profound influence on Emerson's life, but the Philosophers' Camp excursion was a landmark event in the nineteenth-century intellectual movement because it linked an appreciation for nature with art, literature, and philosophy.[3] Most pertinent to this book, the outing sowed a seed in the minds of artists regarding the significance of portraying nature's beauty and serenity as a remedy for the harsher aspects of modern, industrial living. None were more taken by Emerson's thoughts and perspectives about nature than the outing's organizer, William Stillman.

In 1837 Emerson crossed paths with Henry David Thoreau and accounts indicate that the two men became close friends.[4] Ralph Waldo Emerson is considered by many scholars to be the most influential writer of the nineteenth century, yet it was Henry David Thoreau's writings that significantly advanced transcendentalist thinking.[5] Despite being raised in a household of modest means, Thoreau completed a rigorous education, graduating from Harvard University in 1837. Throughout his relatively brief adult life, he distinguished himself as an avid reader, prolific writer, accomplished outdoorsman, and respected thinker. Much of his energy was devoted to exploring the intricate connections between humanity, nature, and the divine, viewing the natural world as a symbol of deeper, transcendent truths. Thoreau's deep fascination with the lifestyles of Native American populations further shaped his views on humans' relationship with the natural world and the merits of living a simple life. Most significantly, however, he was captivated by the immensity of nature and its power to serve as a balm for the human spirit in an age plagued by political unrest, social injustice, dehumanizing industrialization, and rampant urbanization. He believed that communing with nature enabled individuals to rise above the distractions of daily life and pursue higher, more meaningful aspirations.

In 1845, Thoreau built a small cabin on the shores of Walden Pond and lived on fourteen acres of land owned by Emerson. He occupied the cabin for two years, spending his time reading, writing, hiking, gardening, and fishing. His experience living a self-sufficient lifestyle became the subject of his now famous book, *Walden*.[6] From this point forward, his writings focused on understanding life's barest necessities, as opposed to "the mass of men leading lives of quiet desperation." For Thoreau, one of life's most important necessities is good health. In his mind, modern people are living in polluted, stress-laden environments that undermine their ability to maintain proper physical and mental health. The most effective way to combat such dehumanizing urban living is to escape to nature.

Because of his deep love for nature and resolute environmental ethic, combined with his rich descriptions of wilderness, Henry David Thoreau is considered the father of American nature writing, and his name is closely associated with ecology and the modern environmental movement.[7] As a trailblazing advocate for environmental stewardship, Thoreau admonished individuals who forget that humans are an integral part of nature and called upon society to honor and respect the natural environment for its divine connection and healing qualities.

The first year the Transcendentalist Club met all of its members were men. Realizing the deficiency of this gender-segregated space, the following year women were encouraged to join the club. In 1837, renowned journalist, progressive thinker, and women's rights advocate Margaret Fuller became an influential member of the transcendentalist circle. When the group launched its periodical, *The Dial*, in 1840, Fuller served as its inaugural editor shaping the publication's voice and vision. Under her stewardship, the journal featured articles written by most of the notable transcendentalists, addressing subjects such as education, government, law, literature, religion, and the arts. Fuller stepped down as editor in 1844 but remained an active voice, continuing to write (particularly on women's rights) and organize women's conferences. That same year, she joined Horace Greeley's *New York Tribune*, where she penned pithy, thought-provoking critiques of the social issues of the day. Her life and career were cut short in 1850 when she drowned in a hurricane off the coast of New York. In addition to being a relentless advocate for equality and human rights, Fuller also wrote about the importance of withdrawing from the noise and turmoil of the modern world, returning only after the restorative powers of nature had revived and replenished the human spirit.[8]

Although most transcendentalists were based in the United States, one of the movements most influential voices came from across the Atlantic. The English author, art critic, and philosopher, John Ruskin, rejected the march of modernization and championed the interconnections between nature, art, and society. As an early advocate for environmental awareness, Ruskin drew inspiration from his time in Switzerland. He urged artists to spend less time painting historical and religious subjects or formal portraits of the elite, and instead devote their talents to depicting the natural world capturing its sublime, awe-inspiring qualities. According to Ruskin, things of beauty—including flowers, trees, rivers, and hills—are inherently good and an expression of the divine. Viewing landscape paintings and spending time in nature affirms God's omnipotent presence, bringing benefits to both mind and soul.[9] It is evident that Emerson and Ruskin shared similar ideas about nature and art.

Ruskin's voluminous works prompted affluent British tourists to visit continental Europe and experience the majesty of the region's last unspoiled lands, especially mountainous areas like the Alps.[10] His message also inspired individuals in the United States to view the mountains and natural landscapes in their own backyard through a renewed and enlightened lens. With its vast expanses of untouched wilderness, America came to be seen as a modern-day Garden of Eden. Because of his outrage over the dirty, unsanitary conditions of cities, combined with his concern for protecting the natural environment, today Ruskin is considered a prominent figure in the early environmental movement.[11] But, most relevant to this chapter is Ruskin's influence on art, especially landscape paintings. Combined with the transcendentalists' voice, Ruskin's writings inspired European and North American artists to explore and capture (in artistic form) the awe-inspiring, heavenly qualities of pure and untainted nature.[12]

Transcendentalism emerged as the first, uniquely American philosophical movement and offered a new perspective on life and society. Even with decades of hindsight, transcendentalism remains difficult to define and defies easy characterization.[13] There are, however, four central themes that permeate the movement. First, the transcendentalists advocated living a simple, self-reliant life free from the latest technologies. Individuals should think independently rather than blindly follow the masses. Second, the movement zealously opposed social inequality and oppression in all its forms. Third, nature (everything from the majestic mountains and rapturous river valleys to the vast, verdant plains) is filled with divine presence. Finally, and most relevant to this book, the movement focused on nature as retreat, safe haven, and escape from the modern, urban world fraught with distractions and stress. Repeatedly, the movement's most prominent spokespersons encouraged individuals to forego modern living and rediscover the wholesome, restorative qualities of nature.

Transcendentalism spawned a number of related social movements. Building upon the work first started by Margaret Fuller, teacher and social activist Elizabeth Palmer Peabody as well as future renowned novelist Louisa May Alcott emerged as pioneers in the feminist movement, both speaking out for women's rights and gender equality. Likewise, emotionally moved by the same deplorable social and environmental conditions that Emerson and Thoreau wrote about, the modern American environmental movement gained significant momentum after James Fenimore Cooper published three of his earliest novels: *The Pioneers* (1823), *The Last of the Mohicans* (1826), and *The Prairie* (1827).[14] In each, Cooper describes nature as a place of wonder, beauty, and affirmation. For example, Natty Bumppo (a central character in *The Pioneers*) describes his favorite place, Kaaterskill Falls:

> Up in the Catskills there is a place that I used to climb to. There is a fall in the hills, where the water of two little ponds that lie near each other breaks out of their bounds and runs over the rocks into the valley. The first pitch is nigh two hundred feet, and the water looks like flakes of driven snow, before it touches the bottom. And there the stream gathers together again for a new start, and flutters over fifty feet of flat-rock before it falls for another hundred, when it jumps about from shelf to shelf striving to get out of the hollow until it finally comes to the plain. To my judgment it is the best piece of work that I've met within the woods.[15]

And yet, not only do these novels describe nature as an undefiled paradise on Earth, they remind readers that nature is also at risk of wanton destruction. Cooper's work, combined with other literary geniuses of the day helped reshape America's perspective on the environment. As America embraced Manifest Destiny and ran headlong into industrialization, a diverse slew of notable environmentalists voiced their outrage over unchecked environmental destruction. John Muir, for example, sought to convince the public that nature is neither inherently dark and dangerous nor something to be conquered. Rather, unspoiled lands like forests and mountains are places to be treasured and protected for their sublime qualities. The growing synergy among these kindred spirits started to bear fruit with the passage of the Yellowstone Park Act of 1872 and gained considerable momentum under President Theodore Roosevelt's administration. The passage of the Antiquities Act in 1906 permitted the president to set aside public lands for preservation (beginning with Devils Tower National Monument) and laid the foundation for the soon-to-be established National Park Service.

The transcendentalists not only sparked movements in feminism, social justice, and environmental preservation but also profoundly influenced the humanities. This is illustrated by the rich body of work produced by such leading figures as Charles Ives, Walt Whitman, William Cullen Bryant, Henry Wadsworth Longfellow, Emily Dickinson, and Robert Frost. Their most notable impact, however, was felt in art and landscape painting.

The Hudson River School

As the United States came of age in the early 1800s, the young nation sought to forge a distinct identity—one that would set it apart from Europe. While Europe could boast about its rich history filled with castles, cathedrals, and magnificent architecture, many questioned what America had to offer in comparison. With its emphasis on the sublime qualities of nature, transcendentalism offered a compelling answer to this emerging identity crisis. The pristine and unspoiled grandeur of America's virgin lands stood in stark contrast to the pollution and crowding found throughout Europe. More to the point, it was professed that God had bestowed upon this new country such overwhelming beauty and majesty because He favored America over all others. According to the perspectives of the enlightened intellectuals of the era, there was no doubt that America was the new Garden of Eden.

Although the transcendentalists prided themselves in their staunch individualism, they were, in reality, a tightly connected group of progressive intellectuals who frequently gathered in the same social circles, attended the same symposiums, and even took extended excursions together.[16] One such example was the Saturday Club, a subgroup that began meeting in 1855 on the last weekend of each month at Boston's Parker House, where they engaged in stimulating conversation.[17] From time to time, the transcendentalists would retreat to the nearby mountains to reconnect with nature. Alongside these progressive thinkers were renowned artists such as Thomas Cole, Asher B. Durand, Frederic Edwin Church, Thomas Doughty, Thomas Moran, and William Stillman. Over time these artists began capturing America's unique qualities in visual form, using their landscape paintings as a vehicle to promote the ideals of transcendentalism.

Having had limited success painting portraits, Thomas Cole turned his eye to the natural landscape. In 1825, William Cullen Bryant invited Cole to visit the Catskill Mountains with him. The twenty-four-year-old painter quickly fell in love with the 3,000-foot escarpment along the western edge of the Hudson River Valley and the region proved highly inspirational. Cole painted many famous scenes in this area including three versions of the Kaaterskill Falls (the same falls featured in *The Pioneers* by James Fenimore Cooper).

One of his most notable paintings, *The Oxbow* (1836), however, was incredibly popular and appealed to a wide audience. The piece features a meandering section of the Connecticut River immediately after a torrential thunderstorm.* It is a perfect example of Cole's strongly held belief that a landscape painting should be more than simply a captivating scene, it should form a narrative. The romanticized scene depicts the struggle between nature and humans, good and evil. On the left side of the image is a storm-ravaged landscape wild and untouched by human hands. By contrast, the right side shows fields under cultivation reflecting human's efforts to tame the land. It is worth noting that the pastoral scene is devoid of the environmental abuse wrought by the Industrial Revolution. By showing a human-created landscape not ruined by the adverse effects of growth and development, Cole's painting conveys the clear message that it is most

* Since black and white copies don't do justice to the original work, it is recommended that readers search online for color versions of the paintings mentioned in this chapter.

important to respect and value nature, not abuse it. Not only did Cole's collection of paintings reinforce the ideas advanced by the transcendentalists, but it captured the attention of fellow artists including Durand, Church, and Martin Heade. Today, Thomas Cole is still considered the founding father of the Hudson River School of landscape painting.

The Hudson River School was the first artistic genre endemic to the United States. The School grew to include a diverse set of approximately sixty artists, but the underlying theme placed the natural landscape front and center as the main subject of each painting. Artwork produced by the Hudson River School followers tended to showcase the beauty, serenity, and divinity of the unspoiled natural landscape with emphasis on the dramatic use of light. The artists portrayed a sense of place that was uniquely American. Scenes depicting human-occupied lands were invariably pastoral in nature reflecting the innocence and purity of individuals living off the land. To the Hudson River School painters, nature was not only sacred and divine, but was a place of healing for the human spirit. Between 1855 and 1861, *The Crayon* (a journal dedicated to American art) published numerous articles and editorials that focused on the restorative qualities of nature.[18]

The Hudson River School of landscape painting was a relatively short-lived movement in the American art scene, most prominent between 1825 and 1875, with its artists bifurcated by focus and scope. The first generation of Hudson painters not only depicted nature in all its breathtaking glory, but each painting captured the allegory of nature being infused with the divine. Beyond Thomas Cole, Asher B. Durand is the most noteworthy among the first-generation painters. As close friends, Cole and Durand frequently left their studios in New York City and ventured out to hike and sketch together. After Cole's untimely death at the young age of forty-seven, Durand became the leading figure of the Hudson River School. Durand's landscape paintings have been characterized as more emotion-laden and poetic as well as a bit more faithful to reality than Cole's.[19] Durand's most famous painting is titled *Kindred Spirits* (1849). Painted as a tribute to his good friend, the painting features a pristine landscape in the Catskill Mountains. Slightly off-center and standing on a rocky ledge surrounded by lush vegetation are two figures (poet William Cullen Bryant and Thomas Cole) who are engaged in an intense, reflective conversation. The presence of the deceased Cole in this work is particularly meaningful. As illustrated in *Kindred Spirits* and voiced throughout his numerous *Letters on Landscape Painting*, Durand was a man who strongly believed in the personal and spiritual renewal that accompanies an individual who communes with nature.[20]

Another notable member of the first generation was Frederic Edwin Church, commonly considered the most gifted of the Hudson River School painters and one of the greatest panoramic landscape painters of all time.[21] Church's work best represents the culmination of the key elements of the Hudson River School. His pieces capture the love and awe for the natural environment like his mentor Thomas Cole, the romantic element of untouched wilderness like Asher Durand, and the grandeur of landscape painting like Albert Bierstadt. In his later years, Church's paintings moved away from using nature as an allegory for elevating human behavior and instead reflected the fascination and reverence he held for nature in and of itself. Church was so enamored with the Hudson River Valley that he eventually moved his home and studio to a mountainside farm near Hudson, New York so he could escape the hustle and bustle of New York City and be closer to the inspirational, rejuvenating qualities of nature.

Although commonly overlooked because his career path took him into writing instead of art, William Stillman was a keystone linking the transcendentalists with the Hudson River School. After graduating from Union College in 1848, for the next year he studied landscape painting under the watchful eye of Frederic Edwin Church. In 1850 he went to England where he worked under the tutelage of Edward Wehnert. While in London, Stillman crossed paths with John Ruskin and became enamored with Ruskin's ideas about the connections between nature, art, and society.[22] Stillman's autobiography clearly demonstrates that he was deeply taken by the Ruskinian doctrine that nature is divine and inherently good; therefore, spending time in nature and viewing landscape paintings is beneficial for the mind, body, and soul. In 1852 Stillman returned to the United States, continued painting, and founded the art journal, *The Crayon*. In his own words, Stillman writes, "the success of The Crayon was immediate."[23] His personal stock was rising earning him the appellation, "American Pre-Raphaelite." Two years later, William Cullen Bryant (editor for the *New York Evening Post*) hired Stillman to serve as fine art editor of the newspaper. While living in New York City, Stillman met the Brown family who regularly hosted gatherings of transcendental thinkers. Cashing in on his improved social status, in 1855 Stillman organized the Philosophers' Club camping trip where he fell under Emerson's powerful spell of transcendentalism. By the 1860s, Stillman had abandoned painting (taking up photography instead) and assumed the role of journalist and editor at several US and European newspapers. Before shifting careers, however, Stillman was an accomplished painter and member of the *second generation* of the Hudson River School.[24] While he is best known today for his work in journalism, his most significant contribution (particularly relevant to this book) was serving as the key figure linking transcendentalist philosophy with the Hudson River School movement.

Members of the second generation of Hudson River School painters were as highly regarded as those of the first. Two things that distinguish them from the previous generation is their focus on places beyond the Hudson River Valley, and, although their paintings still depicted nature's majestic qualities, less energy was spent on portraying the allegorical divinity of nature. In essence, the second generation of Hudson River School painters were broadening their horizons and devoting their talents to capturing the sublime power and beauty of the natural world.

Few would question that the most famous and prolific Hudson River School painter was indeed Albert Bierstadt. Born in the lowlands of northwest Germany, he emigrated to the US with his family when he was a young boy. One of his first successful paintings featured imaginary views of untouched forest near Niagara Falls prior to the Industrial Revolution. It resonated with Americans who longed for the original beauty and purity of the land. Like other Hudson River School paintings, Bierstadt's artwork enabled viewers to momentarily forget how humans have ravaged the wilderness and step back in time to witness America's nature in its ideal condition.

Although most of the School's artists captured scenes located in upstate New York and the greater New England area, Bierstadt broke with that tradition and instead used his discerning eyes to capture the grandeur of the mountainous West. Commencing with a small expedition in 1859, Bierstadt made several trips to North America's high country spending considerable time in the Sierra Nevada, Yosemite Valley, and the Rocky Mountains of Colorado. Bierstadt painted more than 500 pieces over the course of his lifetime with most being artistic studio compositions rather than representations of specific locations. One distinct aspect of his works is the extreme grandiose scale.† Most of his paintings are so large that viewers who stand at arm's length feel surrounded by the captivating, alpine scene as if they were standing in the very spot where the artists stood. Many of Bierstadt's paintings were featured as "Great Pictures" (a term used to refer to a cinematic-style event where tickets were sold to the public giving audiences the opportunity to witness the unveiling of an artist's single work of art). As the red velvet drapes were pulled back, queues of people would gaze at the canvas through opera glasses and small-scale binoculars enabling them to figuratively step into the picture. Another distinct quality of Bierstadt's paintings is his dramatic, ethereal use of light. By the 1860s, Bierstadt's paintings were highly coveted by art collectors throughout the world. Many of his paintings now appear in some of the world's most prominent art museums as well as the nation's Capitol. In 1998 the United States Postal Service issued a commemorative stamp featuring one of Bierstadt's paintings.

The list of talented Hudson River School painters is lengthy, yet few achieved the notoriety bestowed upon Cole, Durand, Church, and Bierstadt. The paintings by Sanford Robinson Gifford, John Frederick Kensett, Jasper Francis Cropsey, and Martin Johnson Heade, among others, are no less impressive and still command handsome prices. Many of these artists broke away from the Hudson River and devoted their career to painting the natural landscape in other parts of North America, and the world (especially the Andes and the Mediterranean coast). Furthermore, commonly overshadowed by their male counterparts, there were a number of accomplished female painters including Sarah Cole, Eliza Pratt Greatorex, Laura Woodward, and Louisa Davis Minot.

Most scholars who have examined the overlap between the transcendentalists and the painters of the Hudson River School have emphasized how this synergy led to the formation of the environmental movement and early environmental preservation.[25] This chapter, however, takes a different approach. It examines how the convergence of these two movements helped establish nature as a restorative retreat from the pressures of urban life. One of the often-overlooked intentions among many Hudson River School painters (particularly those of the second generation) was their desire to

† Readers are encouraged to search online for samples of Albert Bierstadt's paintings. While digital images cannot capture their full scale, they still offer a glimpse of his remarkable work.

create an immersive and transformative experience for viewers. Through meticulous attention to detail combined with sweeping, awe-inspiring landscapes, their canvases were designed to elicit both intellectual reflection and emotional resonance. These artists wanted to give their audiences a way to experience and commune with nature vicariously. This experience is plainly evident in the works by Cole, Church, Bierstadt, and Durand, but to fully appreciate the connections between transcendentalism, the Hudson River School, and the restorative qualities of art, it is fruitful to examine some of the lesser-known works. Most were in fact completed by second-generation artists.

A first example can be found in the canvas titled *Landscape* (1863–64) by William Trost Richards. Compared to other Hudson River School painters, Richards's work tended to de-emphasize the romanticized elements of his paintings. Instead, he focused more on meticulous, accurate renderings of place. He firmly believed that bucolic, peaceful scenes should serve as a respite from the harshness of everyday life.[26] *Landscape* was painted during the American Civil War. Thus, the canvas provided viewers with a mental reprieve and emotional break from the ravages of war.

George Inness's *Sunset on the River* (1867) offers a second compelling example. In keeping with the tradition of the Hudson River School, the scene depicts the duality of an intense thunderstorm retreating in the background to the left against a field of content, grazing cows bathed in sunlight in the foreground. In the play between shadow and sunshine, it was Inness's intent not only to show nature's unfolding drama, but also to stir deep emotional responses. Critics of his paintings frequently indicated that rather than portraying idyllic views of nature, Inness painted more visceral, contemplative scenes.[27] In 1893's *Sunset*, for example, he positioned a large tree in the foreground that partially obstructs a view of the spectacular sunset in the background. Viewers might find themselves wishing they could walk around the tree. In doing so, Inness composed the scene to draw them into that very spot. Using soft brushstrokes and rich, evocative color, Inness created paintings that invited mental and emotional immersion, encouraging reflection and, ultimately, personal restoration.

By 1900 the Hudson River School of landscape painting was all but forgotten as younger artists turned their attention to other genres, especially French Impressionism. Even Albert Bierstadt's paintings had fallen from favor, and it was not until the 1960s that they regained popularity. In its heyday, however, as a vehicle for transcendentalism, the Hudson River School helped shape American thinking and behavior. Most of the Hudson River School painters (especially the second generation) came to believe that an individual's psychological and spiritual well-being is linked to the sanctity of, and harmony with, nature. Collectively, their artwork enabled city dwellers to escape from life's undesirable, harsh realities and provided them a reprieve, respite, and emotional sanctuary from the ongoing civil strife and conflict. Their paintings gave hope and inspiration to a generation of Americans whose emotions were frayed and whose mental capacities had been exhausted.

In light of today's scholarly insight, it is fairly easy to see that the leading thinkers and artists of the day were encouraging people to use nature as a tool in personal restoration. They perceived nature as a place where individuals could find interest, benevolence, and tranquility (*à la*, Psycho-Evolutionary Theory). Likewise, they regarded nature as a place steeped in an abundance of aesthetically pleasing features that evoke fascination, thus enabling individuals to gain psychological distance from the stresses of modern living (*à la*, Attention Restoration Theory). The next chapter carries the story of America's upper crust one step further by looking at how wealthy urbanites established mountain retreats to escape the unseemly qualities of modern, city living.

2

Vacating the City

Mountain Escapes for America's Urban Elite

The previous chapter aimed to strengthen our understanding of the first major sociocultural force in US history that shaped how nature has been used as a tool to promote personal restoration. It traced the connections between the transcendentalists and the landscape painters of America's first endemic art movement. These like-minded individuals not only moved within the same social circles but also helped sow the idea that nature can serve as a powerful tool for enhancing physical, mental, and emotional well-being. For them, spending time in nature or viewing landscape paintings were obvious ways to find relief (and create psychological distance) from the undesirable qualities of modern, urban life. Their influence was most pronounced among America's affluent segment of society because their activity spaces overlapped and the well-to-do had the time and means to spend their leisure time exploring and communing with nature. It was not until the early decades of the twentieth century that the restorative benefits of nature became accessible to middle- and working-class Americans.

This chapter and the one that follows work together to trace the emergence of places where people have sought refuge from the stresses of urban life and found opportunities for personal restoration. The current chapter continues our look at nature-based retreats favored by America's upper crust, while Chapter 3 shifts attention to the rise of leisure time and the development of restorative spaces accessible to the growing middle class. The story of the Appalachian Trail serves as a natural bridge between the two narratives, linking elite patterns of escape with the broader democratization of access to nature. As expected, elements of the two accounts occasionally run parallel, and at times intersect, creating a rich, overlapping narrative of how different segments of American society have turned to the natural world in search of renewal.

Retreating to the Wilderness

Situated a short distance up the Hudson and Delaware River Valleys, the Pocono and Catskill Mountains have been inhabited for hundreds of years (Figure 2.1). Many of the region's first inhabitants—including the Mohican, Munsee, Delaware, and Susquehanna nations—frequented the region's hot springs for their purported curative qualities.[1] As Europeans began settling the eastern seaboard, the Poconos and Catskills provided vital deposits of timber and minerals used in the nation's pursuit of economic development.* Yet, in September 1753, two naturalists from Philadelphia (John and William Bartram) trekked through the rugged Catskills terrain and their report told of unknown plant and animal species as well as amazing natural beauty. Their narrative provided an alternative perspective on the mountains, one that focused on the awe-inspiring, restorative qualities of the uplands.[2]

As transportation technology improved in the early 1800s, steamships began plying the Hudson and Delaware Rivers. This enabled affluent individuals from the teeming coastal cities to find refuge upstream in the mountains. Members of the Saturday Club, for example, drew inspiration for their writings from their short jaunts to the Catskills.[3] By the 1820s, both the Poconos and Catskills had become popular among East Coast elites. At first, local landowners rented bungalows (one-room cabins) to affluent boarders who sought to escape the sweltering summer heat and congestion of the cities. Located a short but elevated distance from their urban homes, the wealthy then began buying land, building second homes, and enjoying time in the cooler highlands during long weekends and over the summer.

In 1823 the first luxury resort opened. Overlooking the Hudson River Valley, the Catskill Mountain House became a popular destination among industrial magnates, leading government officials (e.g., Ulysses S. Grant, Theodore Roosevelt) as well as many of the era's landscape painters.[4] Six years later, the Kittatinny House opened at the Delaware Gap in the Poconos.

* Although beyond the scope of this book, it is important to acknowledge that numerous Native American communities were displaced as Europeans expanded into the continent's interior, establishing settlements, and designating public lands for national use. William Cronon (1996), *The Trouble with Wilderness*, examines this issue thoroughly.

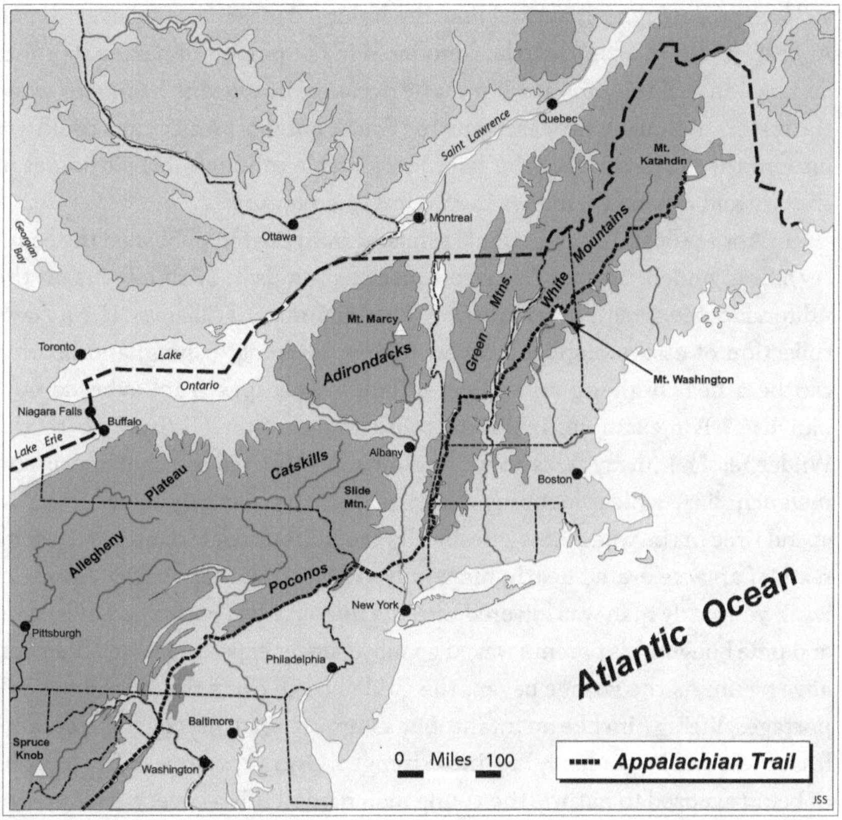

Figure 2.1 Map of Mountain Ranges in the Eastern US. Cartography by Jeffrey S. Smith.

Like its Catskills' counterpart, the lodge's opulent decor was popular among the country's leading citizens.[5] Some people even believed that exposure to the mountainous air would help cure consumption (aka tuberculosis).[6] Located within an easy commute of major urban centers and along well-established transportation routes, the Poconos and Catskills became America's first restorative sanctuary.

Aside from the plush resorts established in the Poconos and Catskills, before the 1860s, the only people to venture great distances into the untamed wilds of nature were explorers, hunters, miners, and naturalists. At the time, leaving the city and spending extended time camping, fishing, and hiking was largely unheard of, and seldom considered. Nature, after all, was filled with vicious, predatory animals and life-threatening dangers around every bend. At best, it was an obstacle to be conquered in the pursuit of personal profits and national development.[7] For many decades, Europeans had recognized the restorative qualities of escaping to nature, but most Americans could not fathom the idea of leaving the safe, comfortable confines of their homes in the city and risking their lives in raw, untamed nature.

In April 1869, a Congregational minister from Boston published the country's first guidebook that changed America's mindset. With a focus on the Adirondack Mountains of upstate New York (Figure 2.1), William H. H. Murray's collection of essays highlighted how hiking, camping, fishing, and boating can be a health-giving and spirit-enhancing escapes from everyday urban life.[8] For example, in his introductory chapter ("Why I go to the Wilderness"), Murray talks about a young man afflicted by tuberculosis and melancholia. As his impending death neared, the man's dying wish was to spend time in the wilderness, specifically the Adirondack Mountains. Despite fears of an accelerated death, his family arranged the canoe trip. After the weak and sickly man was lowered into the dugout filled with a bed of balsam and pine boughs, his parents waved goodbye, never expecting to see their son alive again. As the voyage began, the guide had to carry the invalid over all portages, lifting him like an infant. But as time passed, his coughing became less severe and he gradually regained strength. Over the course of five months of being exposed to nature, the young man made a full recovery. In Murray's mind, the wilderness had received him as a corpse but restored both his physical and mental health.

Stretching from the St. Lawrence River on the north to the Mohawk River on the south, Murray was convinced that the magnificent scenery of the North Woods (Adirondack Mountains) rivaled anything found in Switzerland. As Murray declared:

> It is estimated that a thousand lakes lie embedded in this vast forest . . . gleaming like gems of purest ray amid the folds of emerald-colored velvet. The spruce, hemlock, balsam, and pine yield upon the air, and especially at night, all of their curative qualities. I visit the Adirondacks . . . because I deem the excursion eminently adapted to restore impaired health.[9]

His book became so popular that it went through ten printings in the first year, with the last edition including maps and train schedules from select eastern cities (especially Boston, New York, and Philadelphia). By mid-May, hundreds of well-heeled urbanites had caught outdoor fever and stampeded to the Adirondacks to commune with nature.

What started out as primitive camping in tents and lean-tos, evolved into luxury hotels and lavish estates. The first camp (Pine Knot) was finished in 1879 by railroad baron William West Durant. His modest retreat consisted of two dozen log and stone buildings, a horse barn, and a wagon shed, with covered walkways connecting many of the buildings. By 1885, the upper crust of America's eastern cities had built more than 200 great camps and opulent resorts on the shores and islands of various lakes in the Adirondack area.[10] In many cases resembling Swiss chalets, these secluded summer homes of the rich and famous featured rustic architecture (unhewn logs, stacked-stone walls) and luxurious accommodations (Persian rugs, marble tubs, electric lighting).[11] They were anything but modest. Some of the most noteworthy included, Sagamore (owned by the Vanderbilt family), Camp Bay Pond (the Rockefellers), and Camp North Point (the Carnegies).

In the 1890s, entrepreneurs began building a dendritic pattern of railroad tracks throughout upstate New York, and by the early 1900s, reliable rail service made it relatively easy to gain access to many parts of the remote Adirondack region. Resort towns, including Lake Placid (originally called North Elba), Saratoga Springs, and Ticonderoga, sprang up, catering to the growing demands of the wealthy. During the Great Depression, upper-class residents of Gotham would fork over a whopping $1.50 per person for a round-trip ticket to the depots nearest their estates in upstate New York. Moreover, during the winter months, Snow Trains (e.g., the Saratoga and North Creek Railway) linked New York City with Adirondack ski slopes.

The Great Camps of the Adirondacks are noteworthy because they marked the first time that wealthy Americans began vacating (origin of the American word: vacation) the cities of the East Coast.[12] The Adirondacks became a playground for America's ultra-wealthy and a place of refuge from the pressures and undesirable qualities of modern city living. It was common for wealthy businessmen to send their families up early and then join them during extended weekends. By 1900, the Adirondack region had become so popular that the resident population grew to over 25,000 largely on the economic foundation laid by the leisure class.

The Adirondacks were not the only place in upstate New York that appealed to the affluent. In the early 1800s, Niagara Falls was a "must see" among American, Canadian, and European socialites (Figure 2.1). Prior to the completion of the Erie Canal, a trip to Niagara Falls required an expensive, arduous stagecoach ride through dense forests and over rugged terrain. Once there, however, witnessing nature's power and beauty was deemed well worth the trip.[13] It enabled people to forget (and distance themselves from) the stresses of life. Following the completion of the Erie Canal in 1825, Niagara Falls became significantly more accessible to the public. By 1846, the iconic Maid of the Mist steamboat began ferrying passengers within mere feet of the cathartic, crashing waters. As word of nature's restorative power circulated, the allure of Niagara Falls grew, drawing an ever-increasing number of visitors seeking renewal and awe. By 1880, well over a half million people were visiting Niagara Falls each year and wealthy visitors began complaining that the region had become spoiled by pushy adventure guides and an overabundance of souvenir stands.[14] The well-heeled looked for alternative places to find relief from the noise, congestion, and stress of city life.

Stretching from northern New Hampshire into northwestern Maine, the White Mountains were even more isolated and harder to reach than most other mountain ranges in the eastern United States (Figure 2.1). At first, the region's rugged terrain and dramatic scenery appealed only to the most intrepid and hearty individuals. In 1790, Abel Crawford became the first permanent settler in the area when he moved his family from northeast Vermont to New Hampshire's White Mountain Notch.[15] A year later, he sold the family's modest cabin to his father-in-law (Eleazar Rosebrook) and built a new homestead at a more spectacular location. In 1819, the elder Crawford and his 27-year-old son (Ethan Allen) cut an 8.5-mile trail to the summit of Mount Washington. Their efforts earned them a reputation as the region's premier mountain guides.[16] The trail they blazed (now known as Crawford Path) holds the distinction of being the oldest continuously used hiking trail in the United States.[17]

Over the next decade, a slow stream of settlers began carving out homesteads in the White Mountains, but few people visited the region for adventure or pleasure. In 1826, that changed when an avalanche killed all seven members of the Willey family near Mount Washington. The following year, poets, painters, and philosophers, including Thomas Cole, Washington Irving, and Henry David Thoreau, were drawn to the White Mountains because of the area's raw, untamed beauty.[18] The region became the focal point in the emergence of a cult of scenery (a movement that promoted the appeal of nature's untouched beauty).[19] As a curiosity attraction, the infamous Willey family cabin was included as a stop on the Fashionable Tour (America's equivalent to Europe's elite Grand Tour),[20] but the highlight of any visit to the White Mountains involved hiking Crawford Path to the top of Mount Washington and enjoying the breathtaking views.

Recognizing the region's economic potential, two years after the deadly snowslide, Abel Crawford and his sons built the area's first tavern and lodge at the crest of White Mountain Notch. A short time later, Eleazar Rosebrook opened his own hotel. Over the next thirty years, the extended family of innkeepers and regionally famous outdoorsmen rented rooms at their ever-expanding lodges. After numerous structure fires and changes in ownership, the Crawford House grew to become the largest hotel in the White Mountains; three stories tall and able to accommodate up to 400 guests.[21] To meet the growing demand for outdoor adventure in the region, other Grand Hotels were built in the forests of New Hampshire's tallest mountains. The most prominent included the understated Profile House, Alpine House, Thompson's Glen House, Gibbs's Notch House, and The White-Mountain House, as well as the Mount Washington Hotel. The White Mountains became known within elite circles as the place to go to get away from the city, commune with nature, and achieve personal restoration. In his 1858 guidebook, author John Spaulding writes:

> The world-wide reputation of these mountains *[and White-Mountain hotels]*, yearly calls to their airy heights and shaded sylvan retreats thousands from all parts of the world, that in this mountain land they may for a season shake off the perplexities of business life, and freely received the invigorating influence of health and comfort. For the accommodation of these numerous visitors, mammoth hotels have been erected in the most attractive localities and managed on the most approved city style. Within a pleasant drive of the base of these mountains are places where the free circulation of fresh mountain air, and pure water, afford to all who come and tarry a pleasant and healthful contrast to the sickly, pent-up city street, where floats a hot atmosphere of pestilence and death.[22]

In the 1870s, as many as 10,000 people were visiting the White Mountains in New Hampshire and Maine each summer and by the 1890s that number swelled to 200,000.[23] Despite the steady increase in visitors by the end of the nineteenth century, the White Mountains (like the Poconos, Catskills, and Adirondacks) remained primarily a restorative retreat for the elite. In the early years, it was widely popular for the wealthy to spend the summer visiting various sites along the Fashionable Tour. By the closing decades of the nineteenth century, convention had changed, and it became more common for the upper crust to pass the hot and steamy summer months at their secluded, hillside camps or at an exclusive mountain resort, returning to city life when temperatures dropped in autumn.

In retrospect, Abel and Ethan Allen Crawford were true trailblazers in every sense of the word. They not only established the first homestead in the White Mountains and opened the region's first lodge at White Mountain Notch, but also constructed America's first hiking trail for the purpose of outdoor recreation and personal enjoyment. At the outset, it was the affluent (those with the financial means and ample leisure time) who first hired guides to lead them along Crawford Path to the summit of Mount Washington. As word spread and the trail's popularity grew, it ignited broader interest in replicating the wilderness experience closer to East Coast urban centers. The aim was to offer wealthy residents a restorative experience and an escape from the pressures of city life. Following the Crawfords' example and drawing inspiration from similar European ventures, a growing number of affluent Americans began forming hiking and adventure clubs.[24] By the early 1900s, wealthy residents of most Eastern Seaboard cities stretching from Portland, Maine, to Greenville, South Carolina, could join organized outdoor excursions through hiking clubs and outdoor societies. With names like The Appalachian Mountain Club, Dartmouth Outing Club, Fresh Air Club, Green Mountain Club, New England Trail Conference, Hudson Guild, and the Peoples Educational Camp Society, these organizations created hundreds of miles of independent trail systems.[25] In 1921, land use planner Benton MacKaye introduced a bold vision to unite these scattered trails into a single, continuous East Coast hiking corridor (an idea that would eventually become the Appalachian Trail).[26]

The Appalachian Trail

Deeply concerned about the declining quality of life in modern cities and recognizing the urgent need for urban residents to find refuge in unspoiled nature to restore their mental and emotional capacities, MacKaye envisioned an uninterrupted trail that would extend from Mount Washington in the north, pass through the Northwood mountains (including the Green Mountains, Berkshires, Catskills, and Poconos), wind alongside some of the region's mighty rivers, and terminate at Mount Mitchell in the south

(Figure 2.1). Not only would the Appalachian Trail (AT) connect the two far-flung mountains (about 1,085 miles apart), but along the route would be a series of rustic (yet well-maintained) shelter camps for hikers to use. These camps would be strategically located at convenient distances to allow for a comfortable day's walk and would offer facilities for sleeping and serving meals. In MacKaye's mind, "the Appalachian Trail and the camp community would become a sanctuary and a refuge from the scramble of every-day life."[27] Moreover, the footpath would become the connective tissue between humans and nature.[28] In essence, MacKaye envisioned that time spent hiking the trail and communing with nature would be a respite and sanctuary from the daily grind of city life.

In 1925, members of the various hiking and trail clubs met in Washington, DC, and founded the Appalachian Trail Conference, but momentum quickly stalled. Five years later, avid hiker and successful attorney Myron Avery picked up the hiking stick and ramrodded MacKaye's ideas through to fruition. Acclaimed author Bill Bryson writes that Avery was a tyrant who bullied clubs into producing volunteers for the project.[29] Yet, Avery is also credited with extending the trail an additional 1,100 miles into northern Maine and central Georgia (Figure 2.1). The entire length of the Appalachian Trail (from Mount Katahdin in Maine to Springer Mountain in Georgia) was declared complete on August 14, 1937, without much fanfare. Despite being referred to as the People's Path because about 66 percent of all Americans live within one day's drive of the trail, it is still one of the best-kept secret hiking areas in the United States.[30] Today, more than 4,000 volunteers based out of thirty-one trail clubs and civic partnerships (including the National Park Service, the US Forest Service, and state agencies) maintain the world's longest footpath.[31] On average, three million people hike a portion of the trail each year. Individuals who walk nonstop from one terminal point to the other are referred to as thru-hikers. Of the roughly 3,000 people who set out each year to complete the grueling five- to seven-month trek (2,193 miles), only about 25 percent achieve it.[32]

After having spent months trudging along the Appalachian Trail, Bill Bryson indicates that at some point something magical happens: hikers gain a new perspective on life. The forest becomes their universe because it is all they experience. Anyone who has spent time hiking in the woods knows that there comes a moment when the rhythmic cadence of your boots hitting the ground drives life's stresses away and you look up and notice, with a kind of first-time astonishment, the amazing complexity of the woods, the casual ease with which the elements of life come together to form a composition that is perfect and peaceful. More to the point, life takes on a neat simplicity consistent with the precepts of both the Psycho-Evolutionary Theory (PET) and the Attention Restoration Theory (ART). Not only is the forest a tranquil place filled with elements of intense interest (consistent with PET), but the woods enable an individual to disengage and detach from the responsibilities of life's daily grind (in line with ART).

There are an infinite number of reasons why people spend time hiking in the woods. And there are an equal number of reasons why people trek all or a portion of the Appalachian Trail. Recent research reveals that the majority of hikers on the Appalachian Trail are weekenders (individuals who hike a portion of the trail on weekend outings).[33] These are individuals who reside in a nearby city and escape their weekday routines by spending time hiking in the woods. At a rudimentary level, respondents indicated that the top three reasons for hiking the Appalachian Trail are: fun and enjoyment, warm relationships with others, and being outdoors.[34] After digging deeper, the researchers discovered that individuals found hiking afforded them an outlet for physical exercise, improved mental and physical health, solitude, and greater environmental awareness.

These same foundational reasons are expressed in an open-access blog titled *Why I Hike*, maintained by the Appalachian Trail Conservancy (ATC). From thru-hikers to weekenders, respondents offer a variety of reasons for hiking the Appalachian Trail, including a sense of accomplishment, developing self-reliance, camaraderie with others, and a greater appreciation for nature. However, a prevailing theme among nearly all of the testimonials is how hiking the Appalachian Trail is an escape from the rat race of life and how spending time in nature soothes the mind and restores the soul. As Janene Sullivan writes:

> [T]he list of reasons for hiking the AT is extensive . . . However, each item on the list circles back to a common theme: I want more of less. I want more living, less work, less complicated, and less of being connected. World news that includes tragedy, crisis, wars, and drama, happen somewhere else. The overwhelming bombardment of media meets a brick wall that I like to call "No Service." Unplugged really happens. And, for a little while, I can enjoy just being. That is why I hike *[the AT]*.[35]

A most apropos testimonial comes from Kenny Seagren who writes:

> I hike the Appalachian Trail . . . to change up my scenery from the urban landscape of Philadelphia where I live and work. With all the smells, noises, and buildings, it is a real treat to be able to head north to the Blue Mountains section of the AT, usually for a day hike. It allows me to recharge and think without distraction . . . hiking allows me to escape my day-to-day and ponder in deep thought. Wandering through the refreshing air, I can reconnect with nature and really achieve an open-mindedness . . . As a professional of the built environment, getting the chance to be in the "wilderness" or away from cars and streets allows me to obtain new perspectives of the environment around me and the beauty of the world.[36]

These are just two of the many testimonials that speak to the restorative qualities of hiking the Appalachian Trail. The Appalachian Trail is not the only path through nature that evokes such strong emotions and helps people escape life's abundant stresses and recharge their emotional and mental batteries. In 1932, Clinton Churchill Clarke envisioned a trail that would follow along the highest portions of the Cascade and Sierra Nevada mountain ranges. With awe-inspiring views worthy of Ansel Adams's critical gaze, the 2,653-mile hiking and equestrian Pacific Crest Trail was designated a National Scenic Trail in 1968 as part of the National Trails System Act. The nation's trail system was off and running.

Ten years later, Congress established the Continental Divide National Scenic Trail that runs along the crest of the Rocky Mountains. As the Continental Divide Trail Coalition explains, "the Continental Divide National Scenic Trail is much more than just a line on a map: it is a living museum of the American West, a place to reconnect with nature, and a unifying force bringing people together."[37] In the mid-1990s, enthusiasm for the trail peaked as 12,000 volunteers completed over 1,000 miles of trail construction and maintenance. In the subsequent years, however, interest in the trail has waned mainly because of a lack of public awareness, languishing volunteerism, and a dearth of local support. Extending more than 3,100 miles from the Canadian border to Mexico's Frontera, the Continental Divide Trail is considered one of the most challenging hiking trails in the world. Compared to the millions of people who hike at least a portion of the Appalachian Trail each year, the number of hikers on the Continental Divide Trail is more selective, but their reasons for doing so are amazingly similar (escape from stresses of urban living, enjoy remote wilderness areas, commune with nature, and recharge mental and emotional batteries).[38] Collectively, the Appalachian Trail, Pacific Crest Trail, and Continental Divide Trail are known in long-distance hiking circles as the Triple Crown of Hiking.

This chapter has examined the sequence of mountainous locations in the eastern portion of the United States where the upper crust found refuge from the stresses of urban life. Changes in transportation technology, like steamships and railroads, facilitated more convenient travel thus enabling the wealthy to expand their zone of influence from the Poconos and Catskills into the Adirondacks and White Mountains. Crawford Path emerged as the nation's first hiking trail intended for outdoor recreation. Over time, the well-heeled residents of the Atlantic Seaboard formed adventure clubs and blazed a vast network of hiking paths. Seeking to capitalize on the popularity of these stand-alone trails, Benton MacKaye's vision for a single trail along the East Coast uplands finally came to fruition in 1937. Hiking through the wilderness started as an exclusive outdoor experience reserved for the elite, but the Appalachian Trail helped transform the outdoor activity into one where middle- and working-class citizens could commune with nature and tap into the restorative, health-giving qualities of the great outdoors. Around the same time, visionary leaders began creating places in other parts of the country where the middle class could achieve personal restoration. The next chapter explains how changes in labor laws combined with a new, personalized form of transportation enabled those with more moderate incomes to begin discovering and enjoying the restorative aspects of nature.

3

Restorative Places for the Masses

Labor Reform, Automobiles, and Mountain Parks

War is horrific, but war is also a catalyst for reordering of social institutions.[1] In its 250-year history, the United States has been involved in 102 wars and armed conflicts. Many have had a profound impact on American society (American Revolution, World War II, Vietnam War), but none has been more influential than the American Civil War (1861–1865). The War Between the States and the reconstruction that followed not only precipitated drastic societal changes including the emancipation of four million enslaved individuals, but also ushered in significant economic restructuring. Factories designed to produce weapons and equipment for war were retooled for other economic purposes.

Marked by the end of the American Civil War on one side and the beginning of Theodore Roosevelt's presidency on the other, the Gilded Age (1869–1904) was an era of tremendous modernization. For three and one-half decades, the US witnessed one of the most prosperous times in its history with unprecedented economic growth. Innovative American entrepreneurs amassed vast fortunes by tapping into America's abundant natural resources and capitalizing on cheap immigrant labor. The titans of industry (Andrew Carnegie, J.P. Morgan, John D. Rockefeller, Cornelius Vanderbilt, and Theodore Vail) took full advantage of this favorable business environment raking in earnings at $10 per minute.[2] Moreover, they flaunted their opulence with oversized mansions and great camps in the mountains.

The Gilded Age was also a time of wanton environmental abuse, uninhibited greed, ruthless business transactions, and rampant political corruption.[3] The tycoons wielded most of the nation's political power through bribes and kickbacks, and the formation of trusts and monopolies in key business arenas including banking, petroleum, steel, and railroads.[4] To fill the growing number of industrial and railroad jobs, the US government helped recruit millions of immigrants from Europe and Asia. Civic leaders were unprepared (or lacked resolve) to accommodate the population surge.

During the Gilded Age, nearly half the US population lived in poverty. Enduring squalid living conditions with inadequate housing, unreliable utilities, and poor sanitation, millions of working-class individuals died from pneumonia, dysentery, and other preventable diseases. Worker exploitation ran rampant across most industries. In 1880, the average six-day workweek was 60 hours long, with some assembly plants requiring employees to toil up to 14 hours per day.[5] For working-class households, life was a daily grind of working, eating, and sleeping, with little time for mental or physical restoration. While the robber barons were raking in money hand over fist, the average worker was earning a paltry $10 per week.[6] In short, the quality of life for most wage-earning individuals was grim and burdensome.

As muckrakers began exposing America's inhumane living and working conditions,[7] grassroots efforts at reform led to growing tensions within the country. The ascension of President Theodore Roosevelt in 1901, however, solidified political and social changes within the country. Roosevelt used the White House as a bully pulpit to rebuke big business, introduce environmental conservation, and champion the interests of the laboring class. His reform-minded, social justice platform ushered in the Progressive Era (1901–1920).

Widely regarded as a time of transition, the Progressive Era pitted the forces of entrenched privilege (such as big business interests) and political status quo against the forces of democracy and equality. It was a time when fair-minded Americans sought to use the federal government as a tool to overhaul a deeply flawed economic and social system.[8] In particular, the Progressive Era witnessed the beginnings of women's suffrage, environmental preservation, and consumer protection, but most relevant to this book was progress made in the areas of labor reform and work-life balance. This chapter examines the rise of nature-based recreation as a tool in personal restoration among the middle class. After highlighting the impact of two key sociocultural forces on American society, it showcases the city in the American West that led the charge in taking advantage of more personal leisure time and the growing popularity of private vehicles.

Labor Reform in the United States

Historians assert that the first efforts at labor reform began in England in 1784, when city officials expressed concern about working conditions in Manchester's cotton mills (especially among child laborers).[9] On the other side of the Atlantic, in 1791, carpenters in Philadelphia mounted America's first (though unsuccessful) labor strike, calling for a ten-hour workday. Despite a tremendous groundswell of support from industrial workers, prior to the American Civil War, virtually no progress was made in labor reform, and organized labor remained remarkably weak.[10] Furthermore, during the Gilded Age, attempts to improve working conditions through unionization were summarily and ruthlessly suppressed by the titans of industry, often through intimidation and violence.

In 1890, conditions started to change when the American Federation of Labor (AFL) emerged as the leading voice in the labor reform movement.[11] Through targeted strikes, walkouts, and general boycotts, labor interests slowly began making meaningful progress (Figure 3.1). By the early 1900s, 12 states had passed legislation regulating working conditions (mainly for women and children), and ten years later the number had increased to twenty-seven states.[12] In the years during WWI, demand for laborers surged, resulting in an increase in the average number of hours people worked, especially in industries directly related to the war effort.

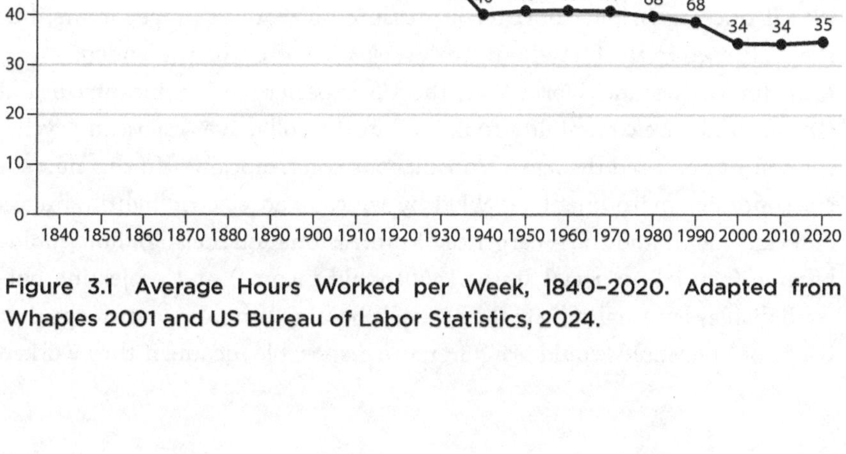

Figure 3.1 Average Hours Worked per Week, 1840–2020. Adapted from Whaples 2001 and US Bureau of Labor Statistics, 2024.

Soon after the First World War, some corporations recognized that change in labor relations was on the horizon and unilaterally began improving working conditions. For example, Ford Motor Company was the first to double worker pay to $5 for an eight-hour day and cut the workweek to five days. Others followed suit, including US Steel, General Motors, Standard Oil, Sears, Kellogg's, and Akron Tire.[13] These corporations embraced a new conventional wisdom. Organized labor (particularly the AFL) moved away from confronting worker exploitation and instead emphasized productivity, arguing that employees perform better when not overworked.[14] Between 1910 and 1920, the average number of hours worked each week dropped from 57 to 49 (Figure 3.1). In the mid-1920s, the argument in favor of an eight-hour workday and a five-day workweek pivoted again. The new perspective held that workers with more free time are more likely to spend their income on consumables produced by big businesses.[15]

During the Great Depression, about one-half of US companies were forced to reduce workers' hours. Instead of laying off workers (leading to high unemployment), the federal government encouraged employers to cut workers' hours but retain a comparable number of employees (leading to high underemployment). This effectively reduced the workday for working-class laborers. When the US economy rebounded and demand for laborers increased again, most economists anticipated that the ten-hour, six-day workweek would return.[16] In 1938, however, President Franklin D. Roosevelt signed into law the Fair Labor Standards Act (the nation's first labor legislation). It designated the federal minimum wage and established the eight-hour workday and forty-hour workweek for federal employees, as well as mandatory overtime pay for individuals working beyond those limits. By 1940, the average number of hours worked each week dropped to forty (Figure 3.1). World War II once again put short-term pressure on workers' upper limits, but they returned to the forty-hour workweek soon after the war ended.

After the Second World War, the US experienced significant cultural change, and a new mentality took hold in the collective American psyche; the country entered the age of conspicuous consumption.[17] In this new socioeconomic environment (enabled by widespread electric lighting, mass entertainment, and the emergence of professional marketing), households became focused on social status (household income) and projecting outward displays of wealth.[18] By the 1950s, it became common knowledge that heads of households could bring in more disposable income if they worked longer hours. This mindset undercut organized labor's efforts to further reduce hours worked each week. As illustrated in Figure 3.1, most American workers settled on the forty-hour workweek (excluding overtime) because it provided sufficient income for a household's needs, as well as enough discretionary money to purchase consumer goods they could flaunt at their neighbors.

For a variety of sociocultural reasons, in the 1960s, women began seeking full-time employment at levels not seen since World War II. To be sure, both the equal rights movement and women's liberation played important roles, but a driving force behind women entering the workforce was a desire to increase household income yet again.[19] In the 1990s, workers began questioning the rat-race mentality and started thinking about a more favorable work-life balance. As a result, the average number of hours worked each week decreased to around 35, where it stands today (Figure 3.1).

Highlighting the changing patterns in labor reform, with particular attention given to the reduction in average hours worked, is significant. At the end of the nineteenth century, working-age adults had little free time, and most of their day was spent doing mundane tasks. For example, in 1880, people spent 85 percent of their daily lives working, sleeping, and doing domestic chores (Figure 3.2). Moreover, when added up over the course of a typical person's

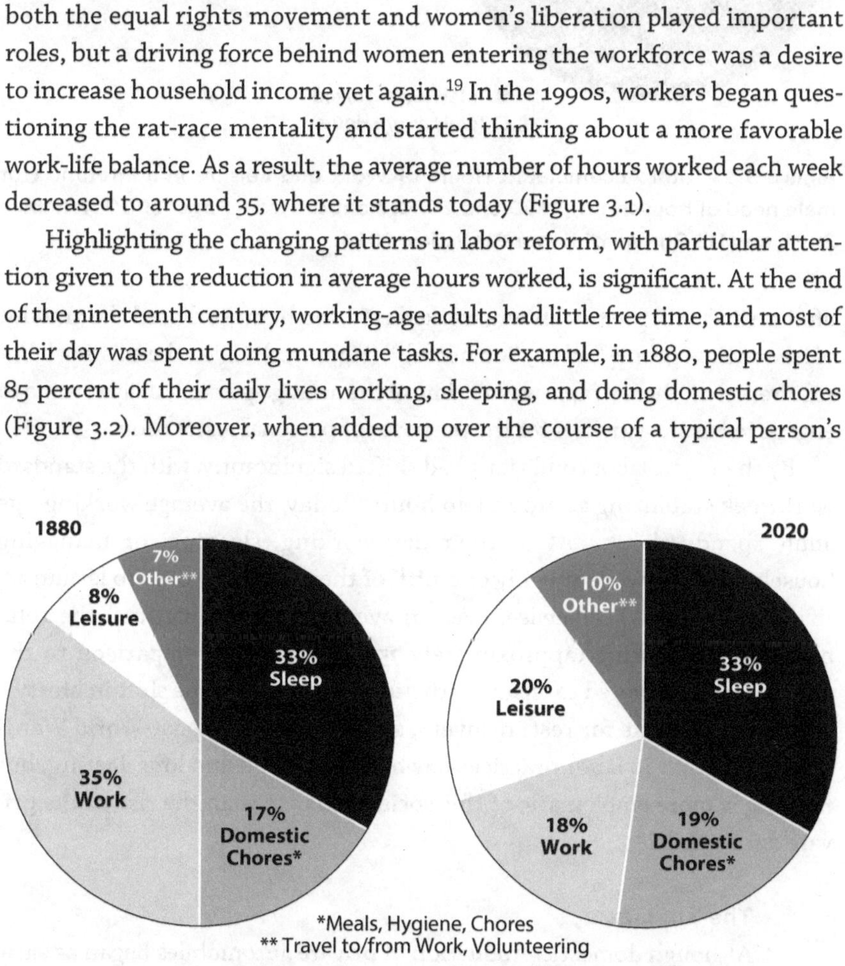

Figure 3.2 Daily Activities for Male Head of Household (percent of day), 1880 and 2020. Adapted from Fogel 2000 and US Bureau of Labor Statistics, 2024.

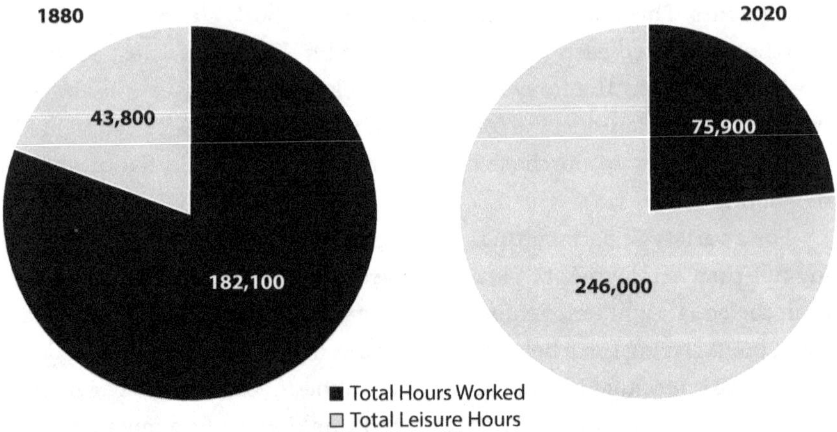

Figure 3.3 Total Accumulated Hours of Work and Leisure in a Lifetime (for male head of household), 1880 and 2020. Adapted from Fogel 2000, Whaples 2001, and US Bureau of Labor Statistics, 2024.

lifetime, in 1880, the total hours worked (182,100 hours) eclipsed the amount of leisure time people had (43,800 hours)[20] (Figure 3.3). Given the existing labor requirements, there simply wasn't time in the average person's daily routine to engage in leisure activities for the purposes of personal restoration.

By the 1950s, labor conditions had shifted significantly, with the standard workweek stabilizing at around 40 hours. Today, the average working-age adult spends about 70% of their day working, sleeping, or managing household tasks, while roughly one-fifth of their day is devoted to leisure activities (Figure 3.2). Likewise, over an average person's lifetime, the total hours spent working (approximately 75,900) pales in comparison to the 246,000 hours devoted to leisure activities[21] (Figure 3.3). The shift in lifestyle affords ample time for rest, recovery, and renewal. The post-World War II transformation in labor practices has been profound and long-lasting, but nothing is more emblematic of this societal change than the rise of the private automobile.

The Tin Lizzie

Although domestic production of private automobiles began as early as the 1880s, in 1903 there were still only 8,000 self-powered vehicles in the United States and less than 150 miles of paved roads.[22] Moreover, the average citizen rarely ventured more than 25 miles away from where they were born because traveling by private car was an activity reserved for the wealthy. When Henry Ford's first automobile rolled off the assembly line in 1908, American society was forever changed. With the simple goal of producing a reliable car affordable to the masses, Ford's sturdy Model T was designed to maneuver over the most rugged roads. Maintaining the same level of confidence they previously held in a horse, people could now take a day trip or an extended outing without the limitations of rigid train or steamship schedules.[23] Flexibility and personalization became the operative ideas of the day.

The Model T achieved tremendous success because it was an innovation geared specifically toward the growing middle class.[24] Henry Ford himself recognized the role that affordable automobiles would play in enabling average citizens to spend time interacting with nature:

> I will build a motor car for the great multitude. . . . . It will be constructed of the best materials, by the best men to be hired, after the simplest designs that modern engineers can devise. But it will be so low in price that no man making a good salary will be unable to own one and enjoy with his family the blessing of hours of pleasure in God's great open space.[25]

By the late-1910s, the private automobile had become a household necessity and it came to define how a modern society lived, worked, and played.[26] Indeed, the automobile has played a central role in countless aspects of American life, including conception and death. From a multitude of perspectives, scholars have examined the impact that mass-produced automobiles have had on US society. With respect to restorative places, ownership of private automobiles afforded individuals a greater degree of freedom as they sought refuge from the stresses of urban living. Thanks to the Ford Motor Company and an ever-increasing number of other automobile manufacturers, working-class drivers could put the noise, grime, and chaos of city life in their rear-view mirror and explore the hinterland, spending precious time in the serenity and beauty of unspoiled nature. A drive in the country became a tonic for combating urban ills.[27]

In the early years, "auto-camping" (pitching a roadside tent) satisfied people's needs.[28] Over time, camping gave way to staying in small, rustic cabins and cottages.[29] Tootling around the countryside became an activity no longer reserved for the wealthy. In 1921, the leisure driving experience was on the cusp of changing yet again when the US government passed the Federal Aid Highway Act, with the purpose of constructing a national highway system.[30] By 1926, the nation's network of all-weather roads was ready for use and America's love affair with cars and driving had fully begun.

US Highway 66 emerged as the nation's foremost road.[31] Extending at a diagonal from Chicago to Los Angeles, "Route 66" passed through eight states and traversed 2,448 miles. "America's Main Street" became a main thoroughfare for family road trips.[32] And as more and more American families took to the road, they needed places to eat and sleep. John Jakle and Keith Sculle explain that by the late-1930s, cities and towns large and small across the country were hosting motor inns (Figure 3.4) and roadside diners.[33] Escaping city life was taking on a new form. As the nation emerged from the economic upheavals of the Great Depression and World War II, the increasingly diverse economy led to the rise of a large and growing middle class.

By the 1950s, ownership of private automobiles had become nearly ubiquitous, with around 75 percent of American households having at least one car, and the demand for transcontinental superhighways was rapidly increasing.[34] In 1954, President Dwight Eisenhower began pushing for a revised Federal Aid Highway Act that would create a national highway system modeled after the German autobahn. Two years later, Eisenhower signed into law a bill that allocated $27 billion for the construction of 40,000 miles (65,000 km) of modern interstate and defense superhighways. The legislation

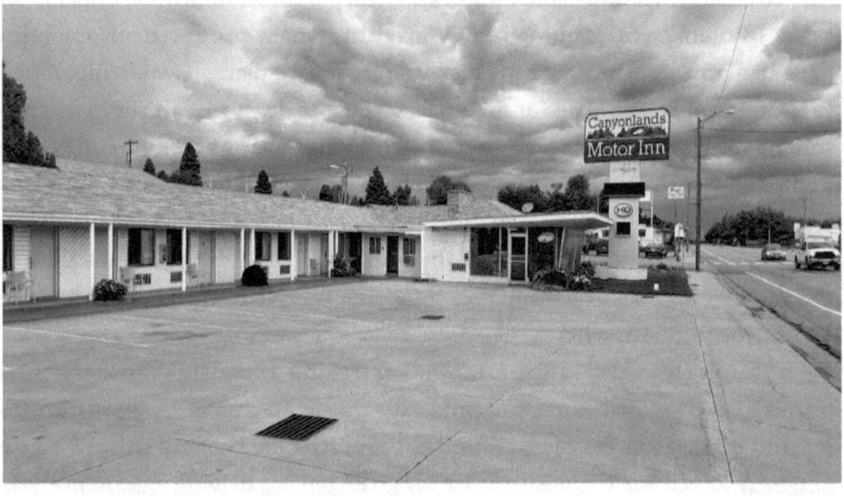

Figure 3.4 Canyonlands Motor Inn in Monticello, Utah. Photo by Jeffrey S. Smith, 2024.

not only provided money for highways, but it also allowed for further construction of roads that gave access to the country's national parks, national forests, and other federally controlled lands.[35] The expanding web of interstate highways and federal roads enabled average Americans to cover most distances with relative ease. To fill their increased spare time, people began taking short driving trips on weekends, and it became customary for middle-class households to pile into the family car on Sunday afternoons and take a drive through the country.[36]

Likewise, hiking through the country's National Forests and visiting National Parks became particularly popular because it was highly affordable and required no special equipment.[37] As more and more people took to the great outdoors, the demand for roadside motels only increased. At their peak in 1964, there were more than 61,000 motor inns saturating the country.[38]

For average-income households, the private automobile gave families greater flexibility, enabling them to travel at their own pace and choose their own destinations. The Poconos and Catskills became widely popular among middle-class urbanites seeking restorative weekend and summer road trips. In upstate New York, the Adirondacks, Lake Champlain, and the rest of the Finger Lakes were no longer an exclusive playground for the well-to-do. By the 1950s, some of the mountainous destinations attracted select segments of the population. For example, when hotel owners in New York City refused them service, the Jewish population took refuge each summer in the Catskill Mountains. The four-county region was dotted with glamorous hotels and thriving small towns, earning it several nicknames, including the Jewish Alps.[39] The private automobile gave urbanites countless places outside city limits to seek restoration.

Not only had the mountainous areas of the East become more accessible, but private ownership of automobiles was directly linked to the rise in the number of people seeking diversion and personal restoration in places throughout the American West.

The growing popularity of the nation's majestic National Parks in the west, including Yellowstone and the Grand Canyon, is largely attributed to automobile ownership (Table 3.1). Even the federal government promoted the region's unique landscapes as places for adventure and rejuvenation.[40] As Newton Drury (former director of the National Park Service) remarked, the private automobile gave people access to a diverse set of federally managed lands (National Parks, National Monuments, forests, and wilderness

Table 3.1. Mode of Transportation Among Visitors to Yellowstone National Park, 1916–1936

	Number of Visitors		
Mode of Transportation	1916	1926	1936
Train/Rail	15,762	40,960	19,472
Private Automobile	13,599	141,644	409,471

Source: Adapted from Weiss 2004.

areas), that lifted people out of their everyday routine and exposed them to new vistas. According to Drury, a visit to the nation's public lands was "literally a spiritual and recreational experience" leaving people remade and reborn.[41] The ubiquitous use of cars was equally instrumental in the success of the Sierra Club's annual trek from San Francisco to Yosemite Valley.[42] Most important to this chapter, however, is the central role that the private automobile, coupled with increased leisure time, played in transforming the "Queen City of the Plains" into a popular restorative mountain destination.

The Nation's First Mountain Park System

In 1859, gold was first discovered along Chicago Creek in the foothills near present-day Idaho Springs, Colorado. Located approximately 35 miles west of Denver, the Clear Creek Mining District became known as the "richest square mile on Earth" with an estimated $1.25 million in gold removed from the area.[43] The vast amount of wealth extracted from the mountains helped fuel a major growth period for Denver. In a few short years, the Mile High City grew to become the territory's most important urban area. When the first rail line finally reached Denver in 1870, its reputation as a gateway community and principal service center was solidified. Thirty years later, as the easy-to-extract gold played out, most Denver business owners turned their backs on the mountains; the city became the region's most important node for agricultural supply, manufacturing, and finance.[44]

As most business interests looked east and away from the mountains standing in Denver's backyard, John Brisben (J. B.) Walker had a vastly different perspective. The savvy entrepreneur envisioned a mountain park system that would attract visitors from across the nation. Regionally famous photographer John Fielder quotes Walker as saying, "There is not a man or woman anywhere who cannot be made over by coming into the dry, bracing atmosphere of Colorado, living in the open air, and forcing oxygenation of his blood by plenty of exercise."[45]

In 1887, Walker and his son purchased the Swiss Chalet Hotel in the sleepy little town of Morrison (about 16 miles southwest of Denver) and within a handful of years transformed the community into a nationally recognized tourist mecca.[46] The center of attraction was a 720-acre mountain park featuring amusement rides, hiking trails, scenic overlooks, musical entertainment, and a funicular railway up Mount Morrison. The destination became so tony that even President Theodore Roosevelt spent vacation time in the Morrison area.[47] The elder Walker was not content, however. His business scheme called for an elaborate system of mountain parks that would attract more visitors than Colorado Springs (Denver's chief in-state rival).

Having witnessed Walker's tremendous success in Morrison, civic leaders in Denver redirected their gaze back toward the mountains. In 1912, city officials commissioned members of the Denver Chamber of Commerce, Denver Motor Club, and Denver Real Estate Exchange to create a system of mountain parks. The newly founded board faced three main obstacles. First, there was no precedent upon which to draw; a country-wide survey revealed that no other municipality in the nation had ever considered the idea.[48] Second, in the early twentieth century, few people in their right mind headed to the mountains for pleasure because the untamed wilderness was still regarded as perilous, not to mention distant and inaccessible. Third, the committee admitted that taxpayers would balk at spending precious tax money on a park system located outside city limits.

Under the astute leadership of Kingsley Pence, the board envisioned a series of rest areas in the nearby mountains where residents of the Mile High City could escape the summer heat, growing traffic congestion, and pollution of the capital city. In other words, places where individuals could enjoy the crisp, clean, mountain air as they relaxed and became rejuvenated through their interaction with nature. As Warwick Downing recalls, "Our conception of [the Denver Mountain Park system] is a chain or series of parks somewhat in the form of a semi-circle. Each park should be connected with all the others by a well-built road, and each end of the chain should be connected with Denver by a splendid [parkway]."[49] Not only would the Denver Mountain Park system become the summer home and retreat for the people of Denver, but the committee saw the network of auto-accessible parks as a playground for the nation, with Colorado becoming more attractive to tourists than Switzerland.[50]

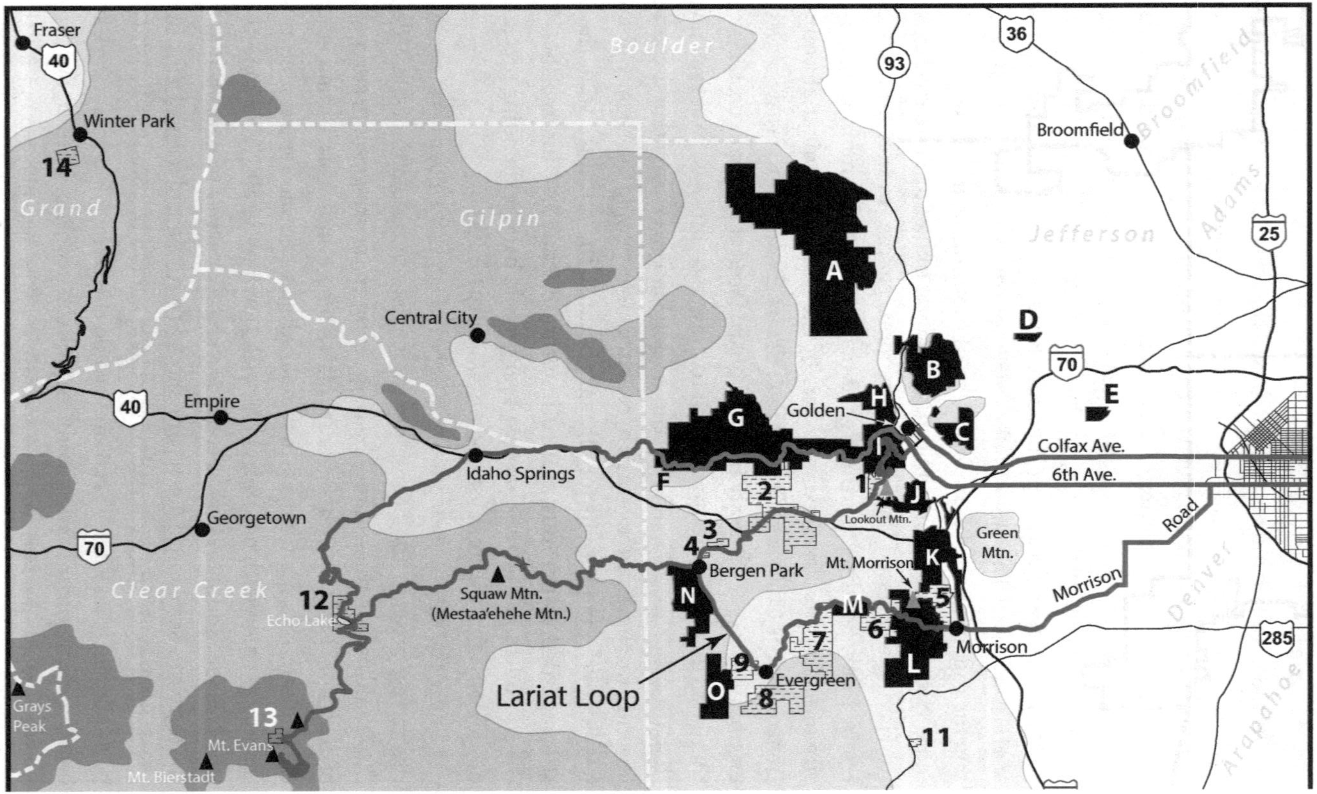
Fraser
Winter Park
Grand
Gilpin
Boulder
Central City
Empire
Idaho Springs
Georgetown
Clear Creek
Echo Lake
Squaw Mtn.
(Mestaa'ehehe Mtn.)
Mt. Evans
Mt. Bierstadt
Grays Peak
Lariat Loop
Bergen Park
Evergreen
Golden
Lookout Mtn.
Mt. Morrison
Morrison
Green Mtn.
Colfax Ave.
6th Ave.
Morrison Road
Broomfield
Jefferson
Adams
Denver
Arapahoe
40
70
93
36
25
285
A
B
C
D
E
F
G
H
I
J
K
L
M
N
O
1
2
3
4
5
6
7
8
9
11
12
13
14

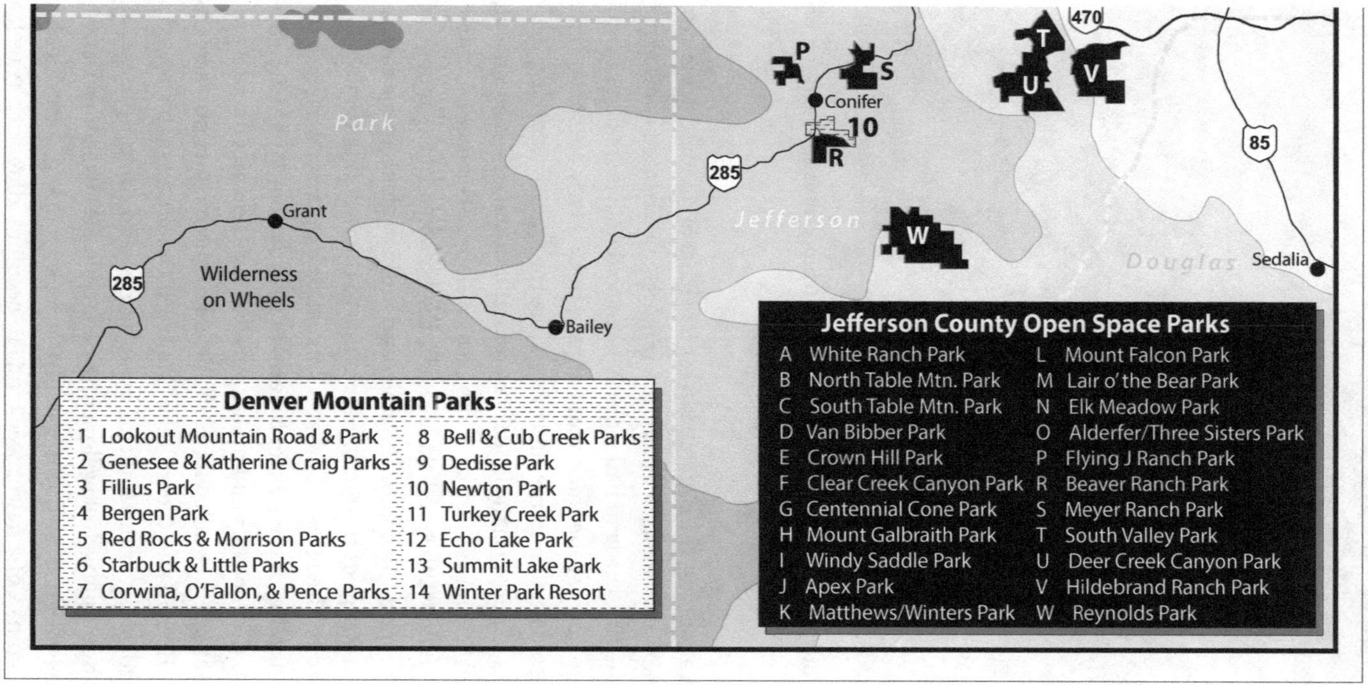

Figure 3.5 Map of Denver Mountain Parks and JCOS Parks. Cartography by Jeffrey S. Smith.

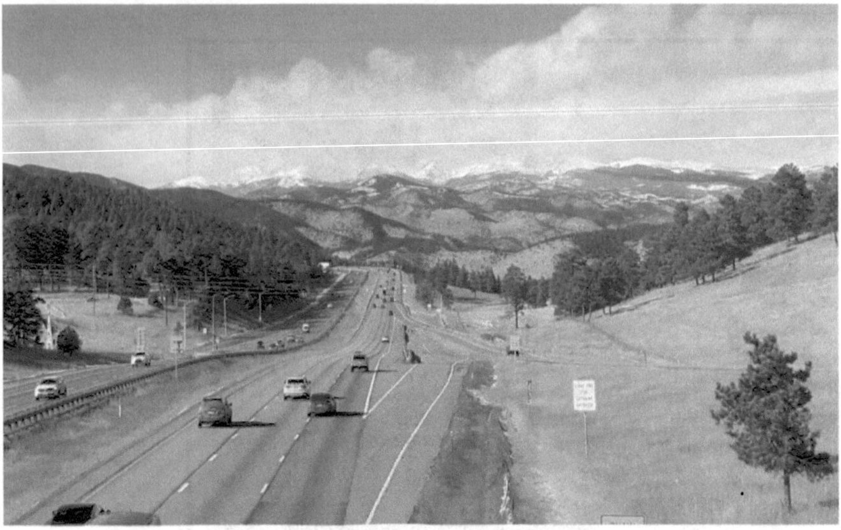

Figure 3.6 Photo of Front Range Looking West from Genesee Overlook on I-70. Photo by Edwin J. Smith, 2021.

The first location that the commission set its sights upon was a 1,200-acre tract of land known as Genesee Mountain (Figure 3.5). Located a few short miles west of the city, the land had recently been sold to owners of a sawmill who intended to harvest the thick stand of pine trees. Many outspoken city residents expressed deep concerns, and in response the committee arranged for private interests to purchase the land for $3,000, thus saving the magnificent, pristine forest.[51] Several decades later, the eastern slope of Genesee Mountain hosted a small, mildly successful ski area, but the highlight of the mountain property was the spectacular view of Denver and the high plains to the east, as well as the Front Range of the Rocky Mountains to the west (Figure 3.6).

In 1912, the city hired Frederick Law Olmsted, Jr. to plan and oversee the systematic assembling of the Denver Mountain Park System. After extensive travels through the foothills and mountains west of Denver, Olmsted presented a master plan that called for city officials to purchase 41,000 acres in neighboring Jefferson and Clear Creek Counties. Olmsted's map showed a network of roadside overlooks, picnic areas, parks, and camping areas, all connected by a 200-mile web of well-maintained roads. He envisioned Denver drivers leisurely progressing down one of the many looping, auto-friendly roads over the course of a day or weekend. To accommodate such travel, a

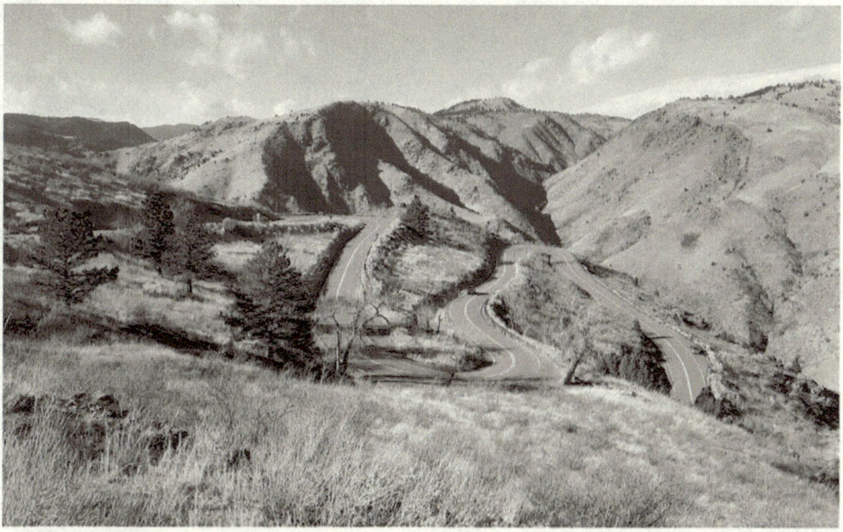

Figure 3.7 Photo of Lariat Loop Switchbacks near Golden, Colorado. Photo by Jeffrey S. Smith, 2021.

generous number of mountainside restaurants and hotels would dot the hillslopes. Olmsted's role in charting a course for the Denver Mountain Park system cannot be overstated. Furthermore, he helped negotiate a land transfer between the city and the federal government. However, when he presented his final proposal to city officials, they regarded it as far too ambitious. Instead, Denver moved forward with a scaled-back ("more realistic") version of Olmsted's plan.[52]

First to be built was the Lookout Mountain Road. The twisting roadway high above Golden, Colorado was completed in 1914 at an eye-popping price of $55,000 (~$1.4 million today)[53] (Figure 3.5). With guardrails on many (but not all) of the curves, the road featured sheer drop-offs and stunning views of Denver (Figure 3.7). In 1915, construction crews linked the Lookout Mountain Road with the Bear Creek Road, and the first loop was complete. The Lariat Loop Trail Road provided access from Golden to Lookout Mountain Park. From there, the loop continued westward to Genesee, Fillius, and Bergen Parks. Then, drivers could proceed to Evergreen and follow Bear Creek Canyon Road downstream to Morrison, stopping at Corwina, Starbuck, and Little Parks (Figure 3.8). By 1918, Denver owned ten mountain parks covering roughly 150 square miles. Each year, in the 1920s, an estimated 70,000 cars

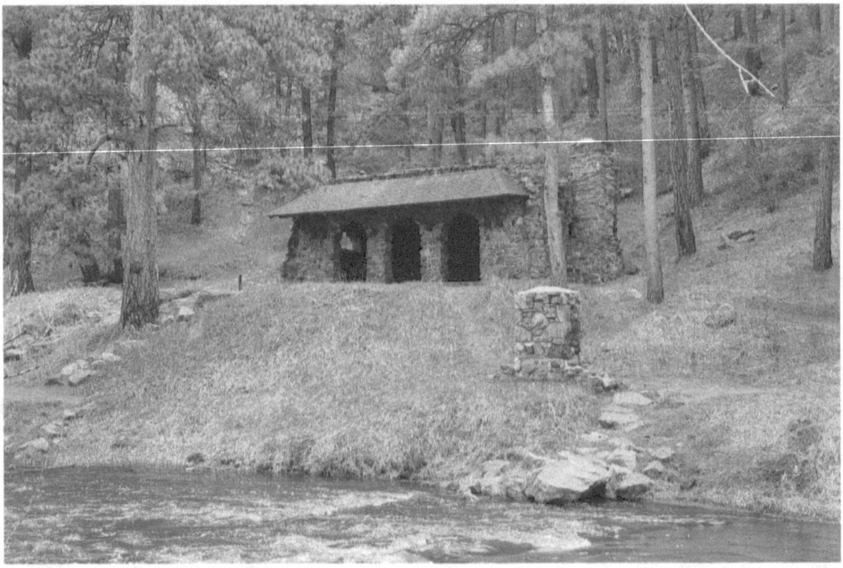

Figure 3.8 Photo of Corwina Park near Evergreen, Colorado. Photo by Jeffrey S. Smith, 2024.

(carrying at least 300,000 people) completed the day's journey between Golden and Morrison.[54] One can easily imagine a parade of Model T Fords chugging through the foothills on a bright summer day.

The crown jewel of the Denver Mountain Park System, however, was the loop that ran between Bergen Park and Mount Evans (the most prominent 14,000-foot mountain overlooking Denver) (Figure 3.5). In 1916, road construction started from Bergen Park up Squaw Mountain (now named *Mestaa'ėhehe Mountain*) toward the base of Mount Evans. By 1921, the road finally reached Echo Lake, and over the next nine years work crews crept up the steep, snow-covered slopes of Mount Evans. In August 1930, road construction finally reached Summit Lake, but it was not until June 1931 that the highest road in North America was open for public use. Critics of the project (including former Denver Mayor Robert Speer) are quoted as saying, "It is a road that starts nowhere, ends nowhere, and never gets there."[55] But even the most ardent opponents eventually came to appreciate the economic and social benefits of the Denver Mountain Park System. Today, a drive up Mount Blue Sky (formerly called Mount Evans) is filled with breathtaking expanses and marvelous vistas. It is still a great place to escape the noise, pollution, summer

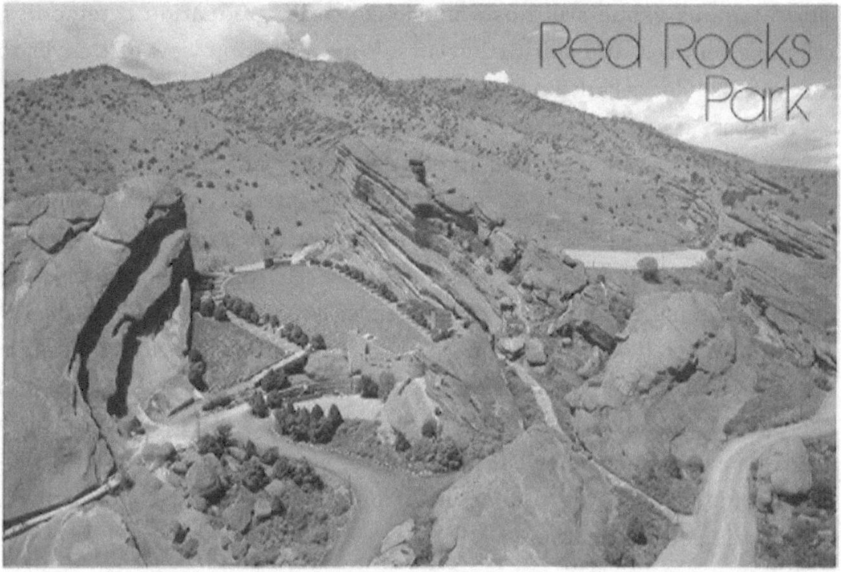

Figure 3.9 Postcard of Red Rocks Amphitheater. Property of Jeffrey S. Smith.

heat, and traffic of Denver. Moreover, during the late-summer allergy season, people drive up to Summit Lake (12,830 feet) to find sinus relief and restoration.

During the Great Depression, the Denver Mountain Park System played an important role in the efforts of the Civilian Conservation Corps (CCC) and the Works Progress Administration (WPA). The best example can be seen at Red Rocks Mountain Park (Figure 3.5). Originally owned by J. B. Walker and his son, the "Garden of the Titans" sat among massive (300-plus-foot) outcroppings of rust-colored sandstone (Figure 3.9). In 1928, the city of Denver purchased a portion of Walker's land situated among a specific cluster of the giant rocks. The natural acoustics of the three massive boulders (later known as Creation Rock, Ship Rock, and Stage Rock) provided the ideal location for an outdoor amphitheater. In 1935, faced with high unemployment and rising poverty, the federal government hired young, single men to construct roads, shelters, stadium seating, and support infrastructure for an open-air auditorium.

Completed in 1941, Red Rocks Park and Amphitheater is Denver's most impressive Mountain Park, attracting millions of visitors each year.[56] The world-famous venue still hosts music concerts, graduation ceremonies, religious services, and spiritual events. With a striking view of Denver to the east, Red Rocks Park is a truly peaceful, picturesque, and restorative place.

In 1955, the dedicated mill levy that allocated funds for the Denver Mountain Park System expired and its advisory board disbanded. Denver's parks in the mountains were folded into the city's internal parks and recreation system, and financial resources for maintenance became overstretched. Despite rising visitation and increasing use, the physical infrastructure (shelters, cabins, roads, trails) at the Denver Mountain Parks entered a period of protracted decline. By the 1970s, a visit to any of the city's mountain parks showed evidence of deteriorating facilities, environmental erosion, and widespread vandalism. As Denver's mountain parks were becoming worn out from overuse and deferred maintenance, surrounding counties began investing money into the protection of open spaces. Most noteworthy is neighboring Jefferson County.

Jefferson County Open Space

Much has been written about the history of urban parks and gardens as well as green space within city limits. Little scholarly attention, however, has been devoted to understanding the Open Space Movement as it relates to peri-urban lands (areas outside, but immediately surrounding a city or town). In this context, open space is defined as undeveloped or lightly developed land for uses other than agriculture.[57] Prior to World War II, most planning professionals focused their energy on creating new parks within the urban fabric. After the war, their attention slowly turned to preserving undeveloped lands on the margins of cities. The budding environmental movement of the 1960s and early 1970s spurred city officials into action. Likewise, the migration turnaround of the 1970s (an era in which peri-urban areas grew faster than metropolitan areas) only increased the demand for low-density residential areas surrounded by ample amounts of nature and wilderness.[58]

With most of postwar growth and development occurring in suburban and peri-urban areas, land conservationists raced against private business interests to secure title to vanishing undeveloped lands.[59] Some local governments across the country started setting aside tracts of land for aesthetic, conservation, and recreation purposes.

The preservation of nature increasingly became an indicator of quality of life and highly desirable cities were defined by the amount of pristine, undeveloped lands (open space) they offered in proximity to residential developments. Increasingly, urban residents were looking for places where they could escape the stresses of city life and achieve a level of personal restoration.

Jefferson County's Open Space (JCOS) program began in 1972 when county residents voted to approve a perpetual one-half cent sales tax that generates revenue for the acquisition of open-space lands, preservation of scenic vistas, protection of wildlife and natural resources, and provision of healthy nature-based outdoor experiences.[60] Two years later, JCOS acquired its first two properties (Mount Falcon and Hiwan Homestead) and began turning them into mountain parks (Figure 3.5). To rapidly expand its network of hiking trails, in 1975 JCOS began its youth work program, hiring teens ages 14–18 to construct and maintain the county's elaborate trail system. Incidentally, in the early 1980s, this book's author participated in the backbreaking, but rewarding work over the course of two summers. Because of an exponential growth in visitation and growing concerns over erosion and vandalism, in 1996 JCOS began hiring Park Rangers to educate the public and shape user activities. JCOS's most peculiar acquisition occurred in 2011 when the county purchased approximately 600 acres that once sat on the Rocky Flats Nuclear Weapons property.[61] The land, formerly contaminated by nuclear waste, now features a lengthy hiking trail that ensures outdoor enthusiasts a place to enjoy spectacular vistas of the Front Range and benefit from nature's health-giving qualities. Over the course of five decades, JCOS has acquired nearly 60,000 acres of land, established 27 Open Space Parks, constructed 966 miles of trails, and set aside 3,100 acres for conservation.[62] Moving forward, JCOS plans to continue acquiring new lands as well as expand its network of trails from its current total to 1,100 miles by 2030 and 1,200 miles by 2050.[63]

As the nation's first sales-tax-funded open-space program, JCOS's trail-based system provides a wide variety of recreational services to individuals of all ages and abilities, including hiking, cycling, horseback riding, kayaking, wildlife viewing, camping, fishing, and cross-country skiing. According to Matt Robbins (JCOS Director of Communications), in 2021 an estimated 8.5 million people visited JCOS's parks.

Recent survey results indicate that 41 percent of county residents visit a JCOS park at least once per week.[64] Through the Jefferson County Outdoors Foundation, in collaboration with Jefferson County Public Health Department, trail maps at each park provide user information on the front side and offer health advice on the reverse side.[65] In 2018, Jefferson County

Table 3.2. Top 10 Perceived Benefits of Open Space, 2020

Perceived Benefit	Percent
Open space for future generations	91.0%
Improves physical & mental health	89.0%
Habitat for wildlife	89.0%
Natural setting close to home	88.0%
Protection of resources/nature	87.0%
Seeing wildlife close to home	85.0%
Place for solitude	70.0%
Improves property values	67.0%
Place to socialize (friends/family)	61.0%
Place to learn about nature	60.0%

Source: Adapted from Kennedy 2018.

commissioned a survey asking residents to identify the greatest benefits of public open space. Among the top ten answers, 89 percent of residents said that open space improves their physical and emotional health[66] (Table 3.2). As part of its Community Health Improvement Plan (CHIP) and Aging Well in Jefferson County Initiative, the county has set a goal of having a public park or trail within a 10-minute commute (walking or driving) of each resident's front door.[67] Jefferson County Open Space plays a vital role in helping the county meet that objective.

Revitalization of Denver's Mountain Parks

As the City of Denver watched neighboring counties safeguard their precious open space and offer places for personal restoration, they realized the importance of revitalizing their own mountain parks. To paraphrase Bart Berger (Founder of the Denver Mountain Parks Foundation), Denver has to get back into the game; it needs to reacquaint itself with the *raison d'être* of its bold park system and join forces with neighboring counties in their commitment to protect open space and natural areas that give people places to play, learn, exercise, and get together, as well as relax and be alone.[68]

In the 1990s, to save the Denver Mountain Park System, city officials petitioned the federal government to list some of their mountain parks on the National Register of Historic Places. This designation enables city officials to apply for grant money that can be used for repairing and restoring the parks'

Table 3.3. Denver Mountain Parks and Conservation Areas Acreage by County, 2021

County	Acreage Owned
Clear Creek	2,780
Douglas	1,001
Grand	89
Jefferson	10,721
Total	14,591 acres

Source: Adapted from Rex-Atzet 2011. Data from Denver Park & Recreation Department, "List of Mountain Parks," (1 January 1955), in DHCP, Box 5; "Named Mountain Parks," in DHCP, Box 2, FF 14; "Donated Areas," in DHCP, Box 2, FF 13; "History of Mountain Parks," in DHCP, Box 3, FF 2. MPAC Minutes, 22 May 1917; 7 May 1918, in DHCP, BOX 5, FF 3, 4. "Gives Mountain Park," DMF (July 1918), p. 16. Gene and Barbara Sternberg, Evergreen: Our Mountain Community, 3rd ed. (Evergreen: Evergreen Kiwanis Foundation, 2004), p. 104. Denver Parks & Recreation Department, "Denver Mountain Parks Master Plan 2008," p. 2.

historic structures and general maintenance. By 2004, benefactors created the Denver Mountain Parks Foundation, and through its efforts Red Rocks Park and Amphitheater was designated a National Historic Landmark in 2015.

Of the 14,591 acres of mountain park lands owned by the city of Denver, most lie within the boundaries of Jefferson County (Table 3.3) and share a contiguous border with JCOS land. One of the best examples is Denver's Red Rocks Amphitheater, sandwiched between JCOS's Matthews/Winters Park on the north and Mount Falcon Park on the south (Figure 3.5). Thus, the custodians of the Denver Mountain Park System joined forces with its neighbor to create a management plan. For example, Denver and Jefferson Counties cooperate to protect natural resources and address growing public use along the 40-mile Lariat Loop Trail and contiguous JCOS lands.

Likewise, in 2008 the Denver Mountain Parks Foundation drafted a Master Plan to help shape the city's efforts moving forward. Among other things, it reaffirmed city residents' continued interest in owning the mountain parks. With a renewed sense of purpose and commitment, the Denver Mountain Park System has a bright and promising future. In fact, for the first time in 82 years, Denver acquired its newest mountain property when the Axton family donated 450 acres to the city.[69]

Created from a grand vision at the dawn of the automobile age, the Denver Mountain Park System was a brilliant plan that took advantage of the relatively new form of personalized transportation and the increasing amount of leisure time that the labor reform movement worked so hard to achieve. The city's impressive park system encompasses lands that represent every life zone found across Colorado (from high plains prairie to high alpine tundra).[70] From its inception and continuing to the present, civic leaders have made it clear that the primary purpose and intended benefit of Denver's Mountain Park System is one of health; economic health of the city and region, environmental health of the mountains and their watersheds, as well as the physical, social, and mental health of area residents.[71] Denver's Mountain Park System is considered one of the city's greatest achievements because it has paid handsome dividends for each dollar invested, done more to promote Denver than any other municipal project, and served as an ongoing model for environmental (open space) protection.[72] The city's mountain parks have transformed and expanded the traditional vision of urban parks and blazed a trail for future open space conservation.[73]

But most relevant to this book is the fact that the city's mountain parks have brought considerable pleasure to city residents by giving them a place that promotes personal restoration and physical, mental, and emotional well-being. Consistent with both the PET and ART theories, the mountain parks on the west side of Denver offer tranquil-rich places where individuals can unplug and disconnect from the daily stresses of urban living. As local Landscape Architect Tina Bishop states, "the fundamental value of the Denver Mountain Park System is having a system that close to home where everyone from every diverse background can participate in a connection to nature."[74] Moreover, regionally famous photographer John Fielder sums it up best when he says, "[The Denver Mountain Park System] puts a park, a trail, an open space, a wildlife area in everybody's back yards so that every child and family has an opportunity to retreat to nature to feel better, not just physically, but psychologically."[75] Chapters 3 and 4 have focused on places where people have escaped outside or on the edge of urban areas. Finding space inside the urban jungle that promotes and enables contemplation, relaxation, and rejuvenation has been considerably more difficult. The subsequent chapter explores some pivotal milestones in US history where governments have created nature-based spaces within city limits that improve quality of life and promote personal restoration.

4

Nature in the City

The Rise of Restorative Urban Enclaves

The structure of American society today differs significantly from that of the early nineteenth century. In 1800, about 94.9 percent of the US population lived in rural areas (Figure 4.1), and their livelihood depended largely on subsistence agriculture.[1] Heads of households owned and managed the means of production, with family members providing the majority of unpaid labor.[2] Although Thomas Jefferson extolled the lifestyle of rural yeoman farmers, the demanding practice of living solely off the fruits of one's labor was rapidly coming to an end.[3] By 1840, the Industrial Revolution had transformed how people earned a living and precipitated a redistribution of the population. Between 1850 and 1900, the number of wage-based factory jobs surged by 600 percent.[4] Young, single men spearheaded the stampede of people moving from the country to urban centers. Mechanized manufacturing offered steady, year-round employment, prompting peasant farmers to abandon their fields and relocate their families to cities. Improved urban living conditions (particularly advancements in public health) further attracted households to urban settings.

By the late 1880s, cities expanded their functions from central places for the trade and shipment of agricultural products to the concentration of industry. American society increasingly became one where individuals produced goods and services they do not consume and consumed goods and services they do not produce.[5] The influx of wage-earning assembly workers led to rapid urbanization, and by the closing decade of the 1800s, nearly 35 percent of the US population was living in cities (Figure 4.1). Some urban areas, like Boston, New York, and Philadelphia, were teeming with people. Between 1800 and 1880, for example, Boston's population grew by an average

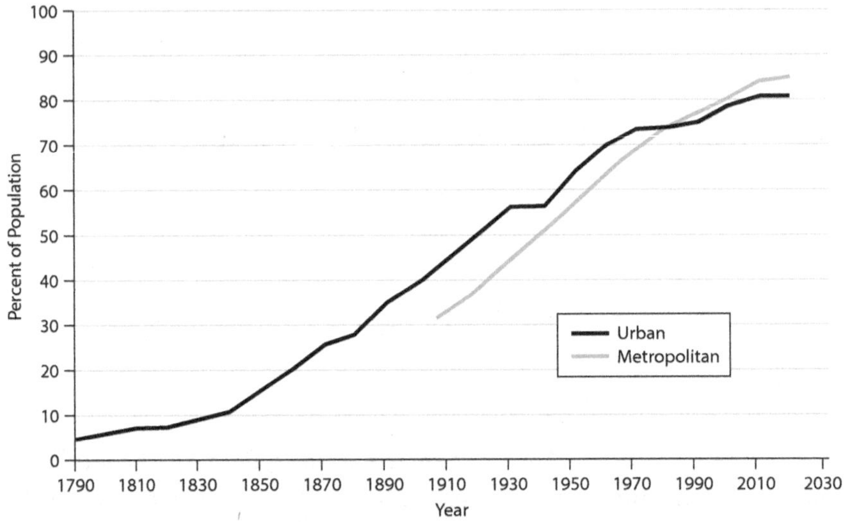

Figure 4.1 Percent of the Total US Population Living in Urban and Metropolitan areas, 1790–2020. An urban area is defined as a town or city with at least 2,500 residents. The US Census started collecting data on metropolitan areas in 1910. The minimum threshold population for a metropolitan area has changed overtime, but it has consistently been referred to as an urbanized area consisting of one or more contiguous counties anchored by a central city of substantial size. The number of metropolitan areas increased from 50 in 1910 to 384 in 2020. Sources: Adapted from Ruggles 2015, Gibson 2024, and US Census 2020.

of about 40 percent per decade, and in 1900 some New York City neighborhoods (especially the Lower East Side) reached population densities exceeding 300,000 people per square mile.[6]

The quality of life for individuals living in these rapidly growing urban areas varied greatly. As presented in Chapter 3, because their position in life gave them the means and opportunity, the wealthy could easily escape the unseemly qualities of city life. For the lesser affluent population, however, their plight was markedly different. As journalist Jacob Riis so effectively portrayed, many of the poorest urban neighborhoods in America (particularly those along the East Coast and near the Great Lakes) were overwhelmed by waste, shrouded in smoke-laden air, and plagued by open defecation in the streets.[7] Furthermore, newly arrived immigrants in these growing industrial cities were often exploited and dwelled in deplorable conditions. The lower classes were confined to these overcrowded, polluted areas in large part because they lacked the financial means to seek respite outside the city. Their well-being rested largely in the hands of government officials and was shaped by the decisions made by city planners. This chapter traces the historical progression of how cities have set aside green space *within* urban settings for personal restoration. It begins by piecing together the remarkable work of Frederick Law Olmsted with the City Beautiful Movement to carve out space intended to enhance all residents' quality of life. Then, it explores a collection of other US cities that have set aside space for respite and rejuvenation. In each case, it is demonstrated that nature is used as a tool to promote personal well-being as well as mental, emotional, and physical restoration.

Historical Evolution of Urban Parks

For the vast majority of human history, people have lived a rural existence.[8] During the Middle Ages, widespread barbarism compelled individuals to move inside walled cities for protection. As the Dark Ages ended and the Renaissance began, Europeans left the fortified settlements and established centers of trade and commerce.[9] Rulers eventually recognized that the random nature of city sprawl, with uncontrolled growth, was leading to congestion, squalor, and disease.

Beginning in the mid-1500s, the city of Paris led the charge in transforming the large and growing population centers. A series of Parisian monarchs (between 1546 and 1870) removed the ramshackle buildings, leveled slums, formalized the street patterns, and constructed expansive tree-lined boulevards radiating out from the city center (*Palais du Louvre*). Emerging as the city's spine, the *Champs-Élysées* came to feature handsome civic monuments (*Arc de Triomphe*), and wealthy estates. By 1600, French nobility created lavish private gardens featuring fishponds, water displays, outdoor theaters, and aviaries.[10] Gradually, these private parks were opened for public use. With its expansive lawns and curvilinear pathways embellished with bubbling fountains, geometric ponds, vibrant flower gardens, and symmetrical rows of shade trees, the *Jardin des Tuileries* is still an outstanding example of a public space that evokes interest and fascination, and allows visitors the chance to escape the hustle and bustle of Parisian city life.

In seventeenth-century England, similar spaces emerged. Inspired by the ancient Roman phrase *rus in urbe* (creating the illusion of the countryside within a city), King Charles II (1660–1685) set aside a dense wooded area known as Vauxhall, featuring walking paths, artificial grottoes, sculptured fountains, and tea gardens for public enjoyment.[11] Likewise, located a short distance from Buckingham Palace, London's residents used Hyde Park and St. James Park as spots for an assortment of outdoor leisure activities.[12] The key to English gardens' success and widespread appeal was their great variety of vegetation. As one walked through the green space, views ahead would unfold as those behind closed. Eighteenth-century British theorists referred to these English gardens as "Picturesque." The manicured English landscape was an ensemble of natural elements (e.g., rolling hills, ponds) and man-made features (gazebos, bridges) used to create an idyllic, pastoral scene.[13]

Unlike their European counterparts, early residents of the New World gave little thought to creating parks and gardens. Instead, leaders focused on moving the fledgling country forward after independence and establishing a solid economic foundation. Moreover, the livelihood of the average American household was still tied directly to the land through extractive activities. Municipal parks would have been of little use to farmers, loggers, and miners. However, the Industrial Revolution was a catalyst for significant population change.

As the new industrial cities grew, some New England urban areas, such as Boston and Hartford, deliberately left green space (aka common) void of permanent structures, ensuring a place for public gatherings and community festivals. Most urban areas, however, became congested places where severe environmental pollution and unsanitary living conditions were the norm. At the same time, America's upper crust looked at Europe's great cities and found their own urban areas lagged far behind in the development of municipal parks.[14]

It was not until the 1840s, when the full effects of industrialization were being felt, that American city officials began recognizing the importance of preserving green space within the urban fabric. They looked to the "City of Brotherly Love" for precedent. Soon after William Penn and the founding fathers established Philadelphia, the municipality began grappling with rapid population growth and a sprawling city. In response, civic leaders mandated that for every five acres of forest land cleared, one acre must remain undeveloped.[15] Other cities, including Savannah, Georgia, Washington, DC, and New York City, saw Philadelphia's success and followed suit in their own distinct way.

New York City's Central Park

Taking a critical look at the city in which he lived and worked, in 1844, poet William Cullen Bryant published an editorial in the *New York Times* calling for a "new park." As Bryant wrote: "Commerce is devouring inch by inch the coast of [Manhattan] island, and if we would rescue any part of it for health and recreation it must be done now."[16] A short time later, well-known landscape architect and noted gardener Andrew Jackson Downing added his voice to the growing chorus calling for a "great park." In 1853, state legislators authorized the City of New York to use the power of eminent domain to create Central Park. With living conditions deemed more polluted and dangerous than most American cities, city officials argued that a large park in the center of the New York City would give residents of all income groups a place to inhale fresh air and be surrounded by trees and greenery rather than filthy, ramshackle apartments, and smokestack factories.[17] In other words, a grand park would be a place where people could go to get a reprieve from the city grind and restore their broken bodies and frayed nerves.*

In 1857, New York City officials organized an international competition to design the city's new Central Park. Landscape architect Frederick Law Olmsted teamed up with his English mentor, Calvert Vaux, to submit a proposal. Among thirty-three entries, their winning design incorporated the ideals of "rural park" and "great park" concepts, both of which called for vast, open spaces filled with natural vegetation. Additionally, any man-made elements, such as buildings, roads, and bridges, should blend seamlessly with the park's natural surroundings. To be sure, Olmsted found in England's picturesque gardens a powerful psychological tool for shaping people's outlook, thoughts, and behavior.[18]

Although the American Civil War delayed construction, in 1865 Olmsted and Vaux took the helm, and work commenced on the 843-acre park. Taking fifteen years to complete, with a price tag of $14 million (~$350 million today), Central Park featured long rolling meadows, rugged ravines, peaceful ponds, and chattering fountains, all connected by a thick network of walking paths. Approximately 20,000 workers moved more than five million

* Paradoxically, the creation of a space meant for beauty and refuge, came at the cost of destroying a thriving community. Seneca Village (a settlement of Black residents and impoverished European immigrants) was forcibly displaced and razed to make way for Central Park.

cubic yards of earthen material and planted 270,000 trees and bushes.[19] In Olmsted's mind, it was essential that the park be ringed with dense stands of tall trees that would screen views of the city and create a tranquil, pastoral setting. Like so many of his other park designs, Olmsted preferred to create spaces that were smooth, bucolic, and naturalistic in appearance. Moreover, there is a sublime quality to Olmsted's grand parks and boulevards that elicits sensations of awe, humility, and solitude. Clearly, a place to escape and rejuvenate.

New York City's Central Park was originally created to give people of all walks of life an oasis from the hectic elements of urban life. And, it has worked. In the 1880s, Central Park received more than seven million visitors per year. Rich and poor alike enjoyed the tranquil setting that sat in stark contrast to the congestion found outside the park's confines. Over time, city regulations and restrictions were eased, giving visitors greater latitude in authorized activities (picnics on the grass, informal sports).[20] Likewise, numerous renovation projects have transformed much of the park into the Great Lawn. In the 1970s, severe budget cuts led to a period of protracted decline and neglect, but in the early 1980s the Central Park Conservancy (a private fundraising organization) stepped in and restored Manhattan's most iconic park to its former glory.

Today, the island of Manhattan is home to about 1.69 million people and its population density exceeds 74,000 people per square mile.[21] Despite being surrounded by some of the highest priced real estate in the world, Central Park is still an oasis for people of all income groups. The 843-acre green space attracts about 42 million people each year and more than 70 percent of those visitors are permanent residents of New York City.[22] Moreover, only 14 percent of the people who spend time in Central Park are first-time visitors from outside the city. The most popular activity among visitors is passive recreation (running, walking, sunbathing, relaxing, reading).[23] Covering a space larger than the country of Monaco, the trees and shrubs that beautify Central Park absorb more than one million pounds of carbon dioxide from the city's air each year.[24] Without question, from the day it opened as the nation's first major municipal park, Central Park has been a prime example of a restorative place; it provides the people of Gotham a space for respite and rejuvenation. New York City's Central Park is but one example of how spaces created many years ago are still helping to make city life more pleasant and tolerable for residents today.

Frederick Law Olmsted's Legacy

Considered the father of American landscape architecture, over the course of his career, Olmsted and his firm oversaw more than 4,000 commissions, including about 700 public parks, parkways, and recreation areas.[25] Some of his most recognized parks include Franklin Park and Metropolitan Park System (Boston); Prospect Park (Brooklyn); Humboldt Park, now Martin Luther King, Jr. Park (Buffalo); the Columbian Exposition, now Jackson and Washington Parks and the Midway Plaisance (Chicago); Belle Isle Park (Detroit); Bushnell Park and the grounds of the Institute of Living (Hartford); and Mount Royal Park (Montreal).

Olmsted is credited with developing numerous landscape design principles, including parkways and boulevards, pastoral style, the necklace system, and great parks.[26] Olmsted's concept of the effect of scenery is especially relevant here. He maintained that the purpose of landscape architecture is to create green spaces that enhance people's enjoyment of scenery beyond ordinary experiences, while also offering a soothing sense of tranquility and renewal for the human spirit. Olmsted intended to design landscapes not as museum pieces, but as places that promote spiritual and mental health for all who visit. He firmly believed that communing with nature was essential for addressing urban, social problems and that naturalistic landscapes could shape human behavior, influence people's thoughts, and enhance one's outlook on life.[27] As Olmsted wrote, ". . . the enjoyment of scenery employs the mind without fatigue and yet exercises it, tranquilizes it, and enlivens it; and thus, . . . gives the effect of refreshing rest and reinvigoration of the whole system [mind, body, and spirit]."[28] In short, Olmsted saw nature as a powerful force for psychological healing and personal restoration. Therefore, the job of a landscape architect is to design green spaces that foster a connection to nature and provide a restorative experience for personal well-being.[29]

In nearly every design proposal he crafted, Olmsted incorporated elements meant to promote healing. In his mind, open, nature-filled spaces should act as an antidote to the tension created by the urban environment. According to Charles Beveridge and his colleagues, "Olmsted subordinated all elements of the park to this restorative purpose. The arrangement of trees, the grading of the land, and the flow of walks and drives all were planned for the beneficial psychological effect they would have."[30] Consequently, Olmsted advocated for expansive lawns interspersed with clusters of dense vegetation. Most of his park designs also included lush plant perimeters.

The dense, towering trees and shrubs formed a visual barrier, separating the peaceful natural interior of the park from the exhausting urban environment, allowing residents a chance to "escape" the demands of city life.[31] Accounts of Olmsted's works indicate that what he found most compelling and impactful in this type of landscape was the abundance of vegetation and its effect on individuals. The richness of plant life created a sense of intrigue, enhanced by the interplay of light and shadow among the foliage. In today's parlance, environmental psychologists refer to this effect as "fascination." This ensemble of landscape elements serves as an effective remedy against the stresses of urban life, providing both physical and psychological restoration.

Frederick Law Olmsted retired in 1895 and passed away eight years later, but his body of work was so influential that it inspired a new generation of landscape architects who carried his vision forward well into the twentieth century. Much of his thinking also helped lay the groundwork for the City Beautiful Movement.

City Beautiful Movement

In the late nineteenth century, American cities were undesirable places to live; the air was laden with coal smoke, waste went uncollected, city streets were covered with excrement, and the water supply was severely contaminated. From a social perspective, poverty was pervasive and uncontrolled growth had led to pronounced overcrowding and crime.[32] The City Beautiful Movement (a term coined by Charles Mulford Robinson) emerged in the 1890s as a response to the growing filth and disorder of industrial cities.[33] Proponents of the movement argued that better sanitation, improved traffic flow, ample green space, public art, and monumental civic centers would make cities throughout the country more profitable and harmonious. As one journalist in 1902 wrote, "the city should be treated as the canvas of the painter . . . to enhance the beauty of any part of the growing city, or to increase its convenience or the comfort or welfare of its inhabitants."[34] A central part of the City Beautiful Movement was the creation of public parks where city residents could connect with the rhythms of nature.

As noted above, given Frederick Law Olmsted's strong conviction that municipal parks enhance the quality of city life, it is reasonable to conclude that his work served as a significant source of inspiration for the City Beautiful Movement. Similarly, as American cities grappled with environmental and social crises, British cities faced comparable challenges. The Garden

City Movement in England provided some cross-fertilization of ideas. The greatest inspiration for the City Beautiful Movement, however, came from the 1893 World's Fair (Columbian Exposition) in Chicago. Held once every five years and attracting millions of people from across the globe, in the early twentieth century the expo held widespread appeal on par with today's Consumer Electronics Show.

Under the watchful eye of urban designer Daniel Burnham, 700 acres of swampland on Chicago's south side were transformed into a model of what a perfect city should look like. Comprised of 400 Plaster of Paris buildings with the Court of Honor commanding a central location, the White City featured all of the latest advances in urban design and engineering, including a sewage treatment plant, filtered drinking fountains, indoor toilets, paved streets with sidewalks, and modern incandescent lighting. Most relevant to this book, the white-painted structures showcased how a well-designed, well-run city could help solve many of humanity's problems as well as strengthen the soul and restore the human spirit.[35]

In 1901, the City Beautiful Movement took on new significance when Senator James McMillan assembled a diverse team of landscape and planning experts to devise a plan for enhancing the aesthetics of Washington, DC. A century earlier, Pierre Charles L'Enfant had been commissioned by George Washington to design a comprehensive city plan for the nation's capital. His vision included radiating avenues, aesthetically pleasing parks, and sweeping vistas, as well as situating government buildings to take advantage of the local topography, notably placing the Capitol atop a hill overlooking the city. Although many of L'Enfant's ideas were implemented and Washington, DC became a cutting edge example of what a Federal City should look like, by the late nineteenth century, officials felt a pressing need to modernize and beautify the cityscape, one more befitting its status as the nation's capital.

With a redesigned National Mall as its centerpiece, The McMillan Plan called for a harmonious ensemble of stately buildings, strategically placed and well-appointed train stations, a monumental bridge over the Potomac, abundant neighborhood parks and playgrounds, and eye-catching public artwork, all set off by attractive fountains and gardens. Throughout the city would be a system of tree-lined parkways that would connect green spaces on both sides of the Potomac and serve as a scenic and recreational refuge for city residents. It became clear that parks and spaces with natural vegetation were central elements of the City Beautiful Movement.

The zenith of the City Beautiful Movement came in 1909 when Burnham and his colleague Edward Bennett unveiled their Plan of Chicago. With a focus on developing a 60-mile stretch of swampland running along the shores of Lake Michigan, the plan called for an extensive network of rail lines and well-manicured grand boulevards, all connecting a necklace of parks and green spaces ringing a good part of the city. In particular, along the lakeshore would be a greenbelt and system of walking trails that afforded city residents an oasis from the hectic and troubling elements of city life. City officials printed 165,000 copies of The Burnham Plan. According to Carl Smith, Burnham told readers they must think of Chicago as a complex system (a living organism) and thus must pursue certain ideals, including efficiency, order, cleanliness, harmony, health, and beauty. Smith quotes Burnham as saying, "The lake shore by right belongs to the people and must be treated as park space to the greatest possible extent. Here is Chicago's one great unobstructed view, begetting calm thoughts and feelings while affording escape from the petty things of life."[36]

During its heyday (1904–1914), the City Beautiful Movement became a crusade against city ugliness as it sought to transform the deplorable aspects of city life into beautiful, rationalized spaces. The City Beautiful Movement gained considerable momentum when its attention shifted from large cities to medium- and small-sized cities (such as Buffalo, Denver, Harrisburg, and Milwaukee). Likewise, city beautification achieved its most lasting accomplishments when its support base shifted from design professionals to middle-class business owners, women's clubs, and neighborhood volunteer organizations. Rubbing elbows with the general public on a daily basis, this population, with its boots on the ground, recognized that most urban working-class people were unable to escape city life and find release from the multitude of urban ills. These grassroots efforts led to countless community improvements. Cities across the country paved and formalized street patterns, installed sewer systems, cleaned up polluted waterways, converted many roadways into wide boulevards, commissioned civic art, and built ornate public buildings. Furthermore, the creation of municipal parks, public baths, picnic areas, and sports fields was a way to improve public health and offer a better quality of life for residents trapped in the city.[37]

Kansas City, Missouri, emerged as a quintessential example of the City Beautiful Movement's success. By the 1930s, KCMO boasted the critically acclaimed Swope Park (1,334 acres of rolling and forest-covered hills), the award-winning World War I memorial overlooking Union Railway Station and downtown, the first shopping district designed to accommodate the use of automobiles (Country Club Plaza), and a network of picture-perfect boulevards. In fact, Kansas City still has the second most number of boulevards in the world after Paris and the second most number of fountains after Rome.[38]

One of the elements of the City Beautiful Movement most relevant to this book is the city parkways. Today, they are a nightmare for the efficient flow of city traffic, but when parkways were first constructed, they reflected creative thinking and lent grace and beauty to countless cities.[39] The tree-lined boulevards with their grass-covered medians, built at the beginning of the twentieth century, typically followed the natural contours of the land and along the banks of waterways. Their meandering design disrupted the rigid grid pattern of existing streets and brought an element of nature into the city. Traversing a parkway gave one the feeling of driving in the country and the irregular intersections made it easy to set aside small open spaces (pocket parks). Furthermore, the network of boulevards and beltways typically linked parks and increased access to green spaces; places vital to the restoration of the mind, body, and spirit.

In the late 1910s, scholars began questioning the logic and effectiveness of the City Beautiful Movement in improving urban life.[40] When first devised, large central parks were attractive and enhanced surrounding property values, but critics argued that the plight of the urban poor would be better addressed, not by large central parks, but rather with green space located in nearby neighborhoods, equipped with facilities suitable for the local population.[41] By the Great Depression, the City Beautiful Movement had run its course and was replaced by a new architectural style known as the International Style. Yet, the City Beautiful Movement has held a lasting appeal; many of the nation's most iconic locations, including Philadelphia's Independence Mall, Cleveland's downtown mall, Denver's civic plaza, San Francisco's Golden Gate Park, and San Antonio's River Walk, owe a debt of gratitude to the movement.[42] The City Beautiful Movement is still an inspiration in cities across the globe today.

Cities are notorious for being places where sensory overload is commonplace. Although some individuals rally in stress-induced, high-pressure urban environments, people commonly find that living in a bustling city where noise, congestion, and the crush of humanity is a drain on their mental and emotional capacity. To maintain proper mental health, urban dwellers need space to recharge and recover. In centuries past, visionary civic leaders in places like Paris, London, and Philadelphia set aside green space where residents of all income groups could find relief from urban stress. The vision that New York City officials had more than 170 years ago is still paying dividends. Central Park continues to serve as an important restorative place.

In recent decades, a growing number of city governments recognize the value of incorporating green spaces into the urban fabric. Cities worldwide are following this trend by setting aside natural space within the confines of their city limits for the enjoyment, relaxation, and rejuvenation of their residents' mental and physical health. Singapore, for instance, has introduced a Nature Pyramid diagram to guide residents in the effective use of nature in maintaining favorable health. These restorative places within city limits play a crucial role as retreats from the bustling city environment, providing locals with opportunities to recharge their mental and emotional batteries.

The next chapter explores in greater depth how nature has been used as a tool to promote personal well-being and physical restoration.

5

Sanctuaries of Healing

From Mineral Baths to Mountain Air

John Muir, the father of America's environmental movement and patron saint of the nation's wilderness,[1] spent most of his life exploring nature. His admiration for untamed lands began at an early age and grew into an intimate knowledge of the natural environment. Later in life, as he helped the US government inventory the nation's uncharted lands, Muir described scenery so astonishing that it tested the limits of readers' imagination. For example, in an 1898 issue of the *Atlantic Monthly*, he wrote:

> All the Western mountains are still rich in wildness. . . . The Sierra of California is the most openly beautiful and useful of all the forest reserves. It embraces the grandest scenery and grandest trees on the continent. No other coniferous forest in the world contains so many species or so many large and beautiful trees.[2]

Muir's evocative prose not only reflected his intense love of nature, but it also demonstrated his fear of losing the nation's unspoiled lands.[3] Because he was so deeply concerned about uncontrolled growth decimating nature's splendor, his primary objective in writing was to convince both the American public and its elected leaders that preserving the country's wilderness was in the nation's best interests. Muir believed that unchecked growth and development were jeopardizing a resource more precious than all the minerals and timber found in the land. America would lose its restorative sanctuary.

Inspired by Henry David Thoreau's writings, Muir appealed to people's self-interest, arguing that nature is not something to be conquered, but rather an antidote for society's ills. As Muir famously wrote:

> Climb the mountains and get their good tidings. Nature's peace will flow into you as sunshine flows into trees. The winds will blow their own freshness into you, and the storms their energy, while cares will drop away from you like the leaves of Autumn.[4]

In essence, Muir saw the wilds of nature as a sanctuary where individuals from all walks of life could find solace and renewal. He passionately believed that a healthy environment was essential for a happy and fulfilling life, and he shared his message with all who would listen.

At the turn of the twentieth century, when infectious diseases such as pneumonia and tuberculosis were the leading causes of death, many health-care providers searched far and wide for alternative therapies that would ease (or perhaps cure) the worst maladies of the day. In hindsight, it appears that some innovative doctors heeded Muir's wisdom and looked to nature for her healing touch. This chapter identifies two pivotal points in US history where therapeutic landscapes were used to treat physical ailments and poor mental health. These locations were part of a broader array of sites that gained prominence because their unique qualities were perceived to promote healing, renewal, and personal restoration.

Hot Springs and Health Spas

Humans have known about the healing and restorative qualities of water for millennia, as evidenced by ancient Egyptians, Israelites, and Hindus dipping themselves in the Nile, Jordan, and Ganges Rivers to cleanse their body and soul. It was the Aegean people, however, who first tapped into the health benefits of the Earth's geothermal waters. The ancient Greeks used pools of warm, sulfurous water to heal skin ailments, relieve muscle tension, and ease joint pain. When the Romans supplanted the Greeks, they took the restorative qualities of soaking in heated water to a higher level.[5] Not only were Thermae (bathhouses) places to gather, relax, and socialize, but centers of recuperation and restoration (especially for wounded Roman soldiers). Spending time in a bathhouse became a central part of Roman culture and the government built the ornate structures throughout its realm. Some of the most noteworthy Sanus per Aquam (SPA) located outside the Italian peninsula include bathhouses in Ephesus (Turkey), Carthage (Tunisia), Malaga (Spain), Baden (Switzerland), and Bath (England).

Geologically, Somerset County, England is known for its rolling hills interspersed with rugged gorges and granite outcroppings. The area is truly famous, however, for its geothermal hot springs, especially near the city of Bath. Oral tradition indicates that centuries ago local Celts revered the hot waters (113°F; 45°C) bubbling to the surface for their mystic and curative powers. When the Romans arrived in 55 BC, they named the area Aquae Sulis (Waters of Goddess Sulis) and by the second century the name was changed to Aquae Calidae (Warm Waters; Bath). The Roman government built a reservoir and an impressive bathhouse that catered to the needs of area residents, soldiers, and workers. When the Romans withdrew from Britannia in the fifth century AD, the baths were neglected and fell into ruin. By the end of the sixth century, Anglo-Saxon Christians had come to dominate the area and St. David of Wales consecrated the hot springs for their perpetual heat and healing qualities.[6] Around the same time legend has it that King Bladud's son was exiled from Bath because of leprosy. The young man lived on the edge of town working as a pig farmer. At regular intervals, the son would take the pigs to the nearby hot springs to wallow in the water and mud. After each visit he noticed that the pigs' skin looked healthier, taking on greater luster. Having stumbled across a cure for his leprosy, the son returned to his father's side and later became king himself. To finish the story, word of Bath's remarkable reputation spread, and the city became an important regional capital. In 1987, the city of Bath and the Roman bathhouse ruins were added to the list of UNESCO World Heritage Sites. Each year more than two million people visit the hot springs in Bath to take advantage of the water's curative and restorative properties. Bath is but one of many towns across Europe famous for hot springs and health spas including the Blue Lagoon in Reykjavik (Iceland), Vichy (France), Baden-Baden (Germany), and Davos (Switzerland). In 2021 UNESCO identified the eleven "Great Spa Towns of Europe."[7]

By the mid-1800s, scientific evidence found that it was not just the warm waters, but the abundant minerals within the geothermal springs that were beneficial for alleviating a wide variety of ailments. Over time two new areas of specialization emerged within the medical profession. Balneotherapy focuses on the treatment of disease by bathing in thermal, mineral-rich waters and hydrotherapy specializes in the immersion of the body in thermal waters for therapeutic purposes. Doctors became convinced that for every disease there was an appropriate medicinal spring.[8]

With the success of Europe's great spa towns in mind, the US government and private investors looked to capitalize on the curative powers of natural hot springs. Places that were once known only to local residents soon became popular health-giving destinations. One of the most notable is a narrow river valley found 55 miles west of Little Rock, Arkansas on the southeastern edge of the Ouachita Mountains. Rainwater and melted snow seep into cracks of the brittle novaculite and chert rocks that dominate the nearby hillslopes. As it descends, the water is heated to an average temperature of 143°F (62°C). After the searing water reaches impermeable bedrock, it is forced laterally to the surface by a fault block creating a series of forty-seven natural hot springs.[9]

Historians assert that numerous Native Americans including the Caddo, Choctaw, Cherokee, and Quapaw regularly bivouacked in the Valley of Vapors to take advantage of the curative powers of the hot springs as well as collect shale for hunting and cooking tools. It is purported that warring tribes set aside their hostilities while in the Valley to ensure that their elderly and infirm had access to the mystic and restorative waters.[10] The first non-native Americans arrived in the late 1700s in the form of trappers and traders who plied the region. In 1804 President Thomas Jefferson commissioned William Dunbar and George Hunter to explore the southeastern portion of the Louisiana Purchase. They discovered several crude huts situated next to steaming springs in the Ouachita Mountains. Their report spurred considerable interest and over time people with assorted physical ailments began gravitating to the hot springs.

The majority of visitors would sit on wooden platforms constructed around the naturally occurring thermal pools.[11] Two particularly noteworthy pools are Corn Hole (claimed to treat corns and bunions) and the infamous Ral Hole (favored by those suffering from gonorrhea and syphilis).[12] However, a few astute entrepreneurs made land claims and built permanent shelters offering added comforts. In 1820, the Arkansas Territorial Government petitioned the US Congress to protect the hot springs for general public use and by 1832 President Andrew Jackson signed legislation creating the Hot Springs Reservation. The federal designation did little to regulate growth and development. By 1870, the hillslopes were covered with shacks while the stream flowing through town had become a cesspool of sewage and trash.[13]

In 1883, the federal government stepped in to restore the area's sanitation and to establish the country's first health spa. Four years later the government opened the Army and Navy Convalescent Hospital for injured soldiers where extended baths in the thermal waters were a regular part of the recovery regimen.[14] In 1892, the first privately owned bathhouse opened for business. What started out as a cave on the side of the mountain, evolved into a formal structure known as Hale Bathhouse. Likewise, the nation's first government-run free bathhouse was built in 1904 to serve the indigent.

Between 1895 and 1920, the US government imposed a series of regulations and funded infrastructure improvements.[15] For example, because of repeated structural fires on top of growing health concerns, the government required all bathhouses to be made of masonry instead of wood. Likewise, in 1901 engineers designed and installed a water collection and distribution system that would preserve the cleanliness and quantity of water flowing from the natural springs. The government's massive beautification project (in 1915) incorporated some initial input from landscape architect Frederick Law Olmsted in its efforts to rehabilitate the area. Superintendent William Parks stated that his goal was to complete "a comprehensive plan on a scale to surpass any of the European resorts."[16]

Under Parks's directives, work crews dredged and straightened Hot Springs Creek and built a neoclassical promenade with gardens along the front of Bathhouse Row. Particularly relevant to this book was the construction of the Oertel Mountain Fitness Trail for doctor-prescribed exercise.[17] Superintendent Parks strongly believed in the terrain cure which held that hiking in nature would elicit considerable health benefits. Because of his convictions, the beautification project included a network of color-coded trails up Hot Springs Mountain with each successive loop becoming steeper and more physically demanding. Recognizing the health benefits of spending time in nature, doctors told their patients that in addition to soaking in the thermal waters, they should walk, ride horseback, or take a carriage ride through the surrounding forest.

As the government made improvements and the Hot Springs Reservation became increasingly sanitary and physically attractive, the number of privately run bathhouses increased. Those still standing today include: Buckstaff (1912), Fordyce (1915), Lamar (1923), Maurice (1912), Ozark (1922), Quapaw (1922), and Superior (1916) (Figure 5.1). Without question, the Fordyce bathhouse was the most opulent, featuring copper-framed stained-glass windows, terra-cotta fountains, marble benches, a well-appointed sitting room, a fully equipped gymnasium, and a rooftop garden. Likewise,

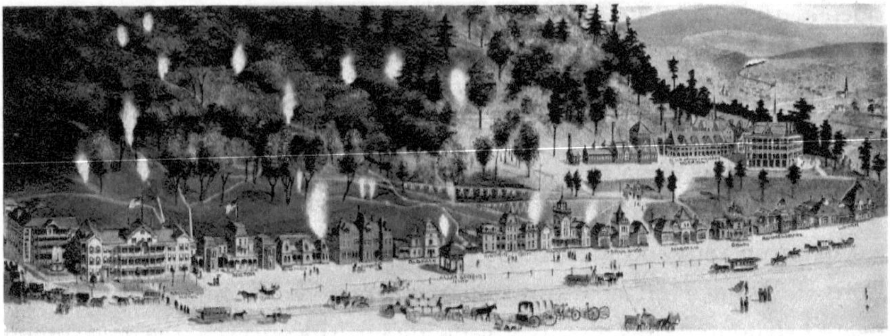

Figure 5.1 **An 1888 panorama of Hot Springs Reservation with the bathhouses positioned in a row along the street. The free bathhouse operated by the US government is situated just behind the row on the right side of the image. Clouds of steam represent the location of the naturally occurring hot springs. Pipes carrying hot water to each bathhouse are also shown. Photo taken of display at Fordyce Bathhouse archives, headquarters of Hot Springs National Park, Hot Springs, Arkansas on 23 Nov. 2021.**

the Quapaw bathhouse stood out because of its Spanish Revival architectural style and the plethora of decorations that paid homage to the Native Americans who once frequented the area. Adjacent to Bathhouse Row, the Arlington Hotel and Baths offered the area's most luxurious accommodations. First built in 1875 and rebuilt after a fire in 1924, the hotel was popular with the rich and famous.

There was considerable variation in the level of services offered at each of the bathhouses, but state-of-the-art facilities boasted the latest in hydrotherapy including hot baths, vapor chambers, needle showers, electrotherapy, full-body massages, mud baths, and mercury rubs. Under a doctor's careful supervision, individuals were treated for skin inflammation, rheumatism, kidney problems, blood disorders, nervous system afflictions, conditions of the aged, paralysis, and STDs. Most clients stayed between one to three months, but some were known to reside for as long as a year. In 1952, the tariff for a single room with bath and toilet at the Arlington Hotel was about $10 per day and each 15-minute bath and massage cost between $0.50 and $0.75. Expenses mounted up quickly, yet people came in droves. Clearly, America's health resort was a financial boon for local hotels, doctors, and pharmacies. Moreover, a robust entertainment district grew up around the bathhouses including restaurants, bars, and nightclubs as well as speakeasies (during Prohibition) and illegal gambling.[18]

In 1921, Hot Springs was converted from a Federal Reservation to a National Park for its historic and cultural significance. America had its first official health resort and spa, and tourist brochures called it the Baden of America.[19] The wealthy no longer had to fly to Europe; there was a world-class restorative resort in their own backyard. Many of America's leading citizens (President Herbert Hoover, Andrew Carnegie, Helen Keller), Hollywood stars (Marilyn Monroe, Mary Pickford, Will Rogers), and famous athletes (Babe Ruth, Joe DiMaggio, Cy Young, Jack Dempsey) frequented the thermal waters. Between the late 1880s and the mid-1940s, a growing number of Major League Baseball teams held spring training in Hot Springs, Arkansas so that players could ease their pain and joints after an arduous day on the baseball diamond. Even some of the most notorious criminals of the day (Al Capone, Jesse James) regularly cast dark shadows on the streets of Hot Springs. But it was not just the rich and famous who visited Hot Springs; people of all walks of life took advantage of the curative waters.

During its heyday after World War II and into the 1950s, Hot Springs National Park was one of the country's most popular vacation destinations. In 1947, visitors chalked up more than one billion baths in a single year.[20] Hot Springs, Arkansas became a mecca for health, healing, and personal restoration. Travel guides and advertisements at the time lauded the miraculous, restorative qualities of America's Spa by showcasing to the public that, individuals would arrive crippled with pain and discomfort and leave feeling healthy and fully restored (Figure 5.2). But also relevant to this book is that Hot Springs National Park served as an oasis from the mundane elements of everyday life; a place to recharge mental and emotional capacities. As the National Park Service tourist brochure indicates:

> A visit to the hot springs was designed to treat not just the body but the mind and spirit as well. Visitors bathed in the thermal water and received massages and other therapies, including mercury rubs. Afterwards, they could relax, drink spring water, exercise in well-appointed gyms, or hike a series of fitness trails.[21]

Despite the widespread appeal and purported health benefits of soaking in thermal hot springs, the mineral-rich waters did nothing to cure the

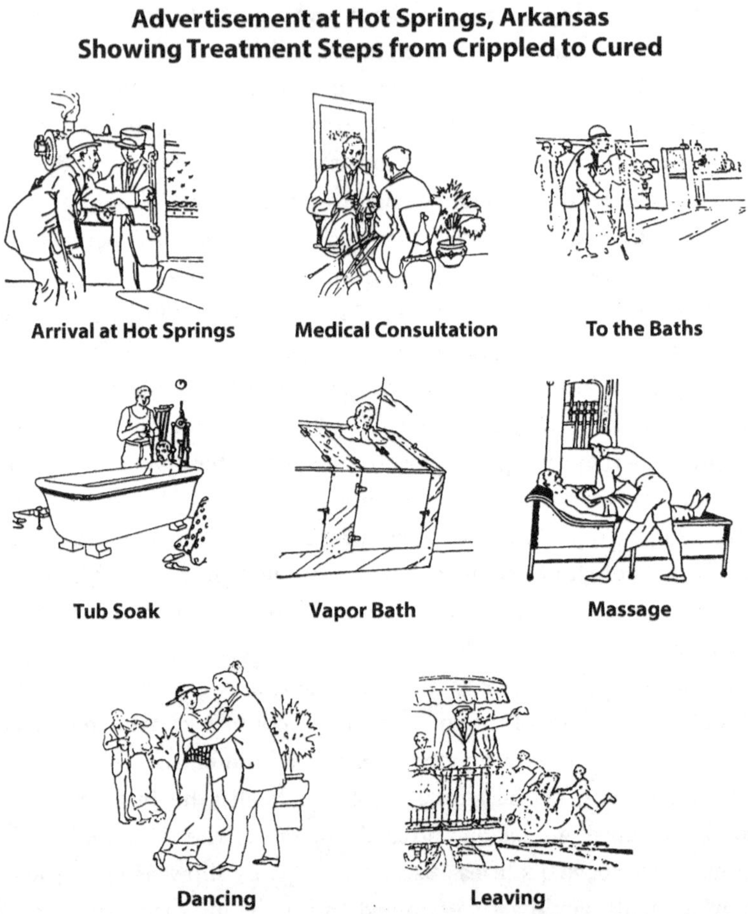

Figure 5.2 An 1847 advertisement showing treatment steps at a Hot Springs bathhouse. From top left to bottom right the images show a man arriving crippled, receiving treatment, and leaving cured. Adapted from a photo taken of display at Fordyce Bathhouse archives, headquarters of Hot Springs National Park, Hot Springs, Arkansas on 23 Nov. 2021.

nation's number one killer, tuberculosis. Indeed, moist, humid conditions only serve to aggravate the symptoms associated with TB. Therefore, lungers (people who suffer from what medical professionals at the time called pulmonary consumption) searched for places with clean, dry air that would help ease their breathing.

Nature as a "Cure" for Tuberculosis

Archaeological evidence indicates that tuberculosis has been plaguing humankind for millennia.[22] Thousands of ancient Greeks suffered from the disease they called phthisis. Beginning in the Middle Ages, outbreaks of TB ebbed and flowed as the disease swept across Europe. In the eighteenth and nineteenth centuries, the malady killed countless people earning the nickname The White Plaque because of how pale an individual would become. By the early 1800s, waves of European immigrants had brought TB with them to the United States and consumption became the country's leading cause of death (more than 25 percent of all deaths).[23] It was not until 1882 when Dr. Robert Koch isolated the tubercle bacillus that health professionals understood how the disease is transmitted. The widespread availability of antibiotics in the 1950s finally enabled health officials to tackle tuberculosis outbreaks. Until that time, however, patients were commonly quarantined and treated in a sanatorium.

The world's first modern sanatorium was built by Dr. George Bodington in 1836 near Birmingham, England. Instead of locking patients in an airtight room as conventional medical wisdom dictated, his line of treatment called for plenty of fresh air including early morning walks or rides and other outdoor physical activity. At the time however, the efficacy of Bodington's therapeutic approach was widely questioned by the medical community.[24] A turning point came about ten years later when German doctor, Dr. Hermann Brehmer achieved some remarkable results.[25] Brehmer's contemporary Alexander von Humboldt told him that pulmonary consumption did not exist among villagers living high in the Andes Mountains. Drawing upon this information, Brehmer moved to the Himalayas and cured himself of tuberculosis through rigorous physical exercise, hearty meals, ice-cold showers in the forest, and abundant mountain air. In 1854, he moved back to Europe and built a 40-bed sanatorium in the highlands of southwest Poland. By 1869, he had treated 958 TB patients with a remarkably low death rate of 4.8 percent.[26]

As word of Brehmer's tremendous success spread, similar facilities were built elsewhere in the European highlands (in many cases, near mineral hot springs), but the hub of sanatoria was Switzerland. The new line of thinking asserted that treating a patient at 2,200 feet (670 meters) above sea level was optimal because barometric pressure and the pressure of the blood vessels were at equilibrium.[27] The new therapy exposed patients to abundant amounts of physical activity at high elevation, fresh air, and proper nutrition. These three ingredients offered patients their best chance for remission, if not full recovery.

In 1875, Joseph Gleitsmann built America's first TB sanatorium on the slopes of the Appalachian Mountains in Asheville, North Carolina.[28] Nine years later Edward Livingston Trudeau opened the nation's second facility in the Adirondack Mountains near Saranac, New York.[29] By 1900 there were 34 sanatoria across the country caring for up to 4,500 patients and in 1925 that number grew to 536 sanatoria with tens of thousands of beds.[30] When the US government finally began formally collecting data on tuberculosis cases in 1953, the number of TB facilities had increased to 839 providing therapy to as many as 136,000 individuals.[31] Many of the sanatoria were in the Sunbelt States of California, Arizona, New Mexico, Colorado, and Texas (Figure 5.3).

Although health providers established sanatoria throughout the country, they preferred locations with the essential climatic factors of dry air, abundant sunshine, and warm temperatures. At a Boston Medical Conference in 1888, Dr. Frederick Knight pronounced that the mountainous West is the optimal place to cure pulmonary consumption because the rarefied air increases respiratory activity. In accordance with this line of thinking, any amount of physical activity at high elevation increases one's heart rate and lung activity allowing refreshing, pure air to penetrate more deeply into the lungs thus enabling greater healing. As John Harner eloquently states, "the intent of the sanatorium was to liberate patients from the disease and restore them to a productive life. The cure would come from the patient's own natural resistance through the recuperative power of nature."[32]

When the Southern Pacific Railroad met the Atchison, Topeka, and Santa Fe Railroad in 1881, linking Kansas City with Los Angeles, people from all walks of life had an alternative route across the country. The new southern transcontinental rail line enabled hundreds of thousands of individuals to head west. Many people gravitated to coastal southern California because of its desirable Mediterranean climate. Estimates suggest that one-fourth of all migrants (nearly 750,000 people) who moved west in the late nineteenth century did so for health-related reasons.[33] Over time, word spread that the desert southwest also possessed a choice climate for people suffering from tuberculosis. Doctors began sending their sickest patients to the sun-drenched lands to capitalize on the climate cure.[34] The cities of

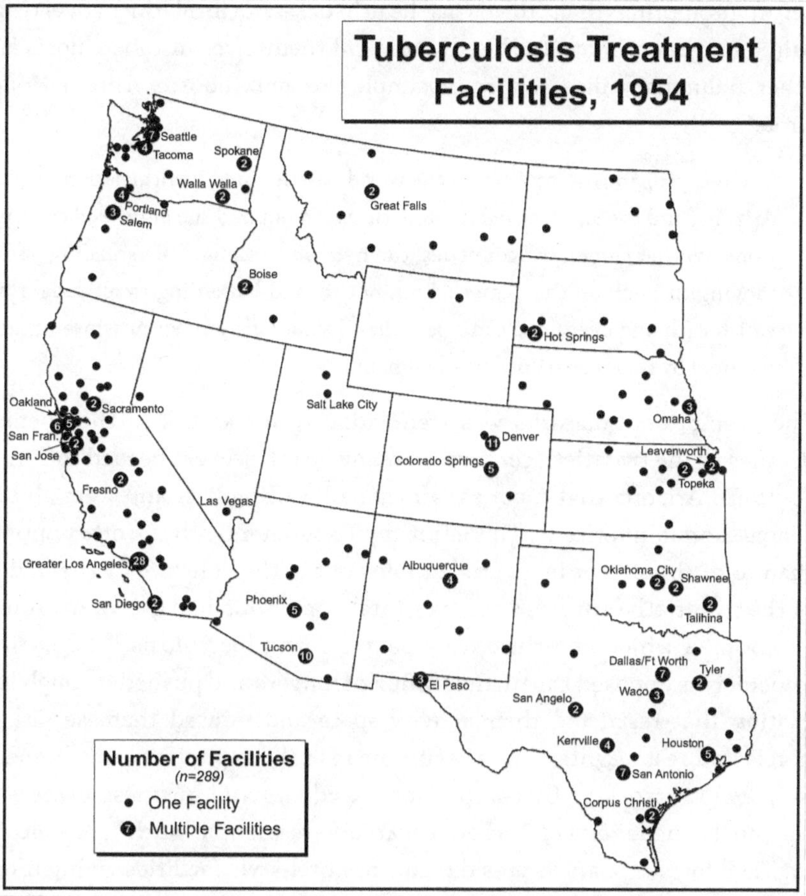

Figure 5.3 Map of Tuberculosis Treatment Facilities, 1954. Data Source: Glaser and Johnston 1954. Cartography by Jeffrey S. Smith.

Albuquerque, Phoenix, San Diego, San Antonio, and Tucson owe most of their early population growth to the influx of people seeking restoration from consumption.[35]

The chronicle of sanatoria in Arizona (especially Phoenix and Tucson) is remarkably consistent. Situated in the Sonoran Desert, southern Arizona is blessed with dry air, warm temperatures, and abundant sunshine. As the surge of health seekers began moving west, local entrepreneurs saw lucrative business opportunities if they could attract their share of the stream of new residents. In the early 1880s, power brokers throughout the territory began promoting their towns as health oases. Scintillating advertising baited lungers to move to the desert to rid themselves of tuberculosis and other pulmonary diseases. For example, Phoenix booster Hiram Hodge wrote:

> There is probably no country in the world with a purer, healthier climate than Arizona, and the sick, the debilitated, the worn out and the enfeebled constitutions of other climes and countries, can here find a climate of exceeding purity, ranging through all the degrees from hot to cold, according to altitude, from which each and every one can select their locality in summer or winter, that is required by their constitutions or ailments.[36]

The promotional material was tremendously successful. In the opening decades of the twentieth century, so many health seekers headed to sunny, southern Arizona that most sanatoria had waiting lists and were able to charge exorbitant prices.[37] This left many TB sufferers with few other options than to pitch tents or build crude cabins out in the desert.[38] By the middle of the twentieth century, Phoenix's total population had grown to around 100,000, of which one-third were people with tuberculosis.[39] Long-time Phoenicians opposed the further influx of lungers and pushed through legislation that restricted their activity space and refused them service at hotels and restaurants.[40] As a result, in 1954 the capital city was home to only five sanatoria.[41] By comparison, residents and business owners in the much smaller city of Tucson (ca. 40,000 residents) were more welcoming. The former Spanish presidio had 10 hotel-style facilities giving it one of the highest per capita number of sanatoria beds in the nation.[42] The Tucson sanatoria operated until advances in modern medicine rendered them unnecessary.

The list of places in the American West deemed favorable for treating pulmonary consumption was long. However, physicians considered Colorado's climate superior. Not only does the Centennial State have an arid environment with fresh air and plenty of warm, sunny days, but the western half of the state stood out because of its high elevation. Indeed, the thin, dry air was known to retard the spread of TB within the lungs. Furthermore, when places like Phoenix, Albuquerque and San Antonio become sweltering hot in the summer, the temperatures in most of Colorado remain comfortable. After his trip west, American Diplomat and travel reporter Lewis M. Iddings wrote:

> The summers . . . begin about the first of June [and are] as fine as possible. . . . Autumn weather and a great part of winter are as perfect as the best golden days of October in the East. . . . The sufferer from diseased lungs has no need to fear. What he requires is dryness, and an altitude which makes the healthy lung do work enough for two, in a place where he is able to lead an out-of-door life, and is never enervated with heat or depressed with humidity. There is, therefore, . . . no better place on earth for the sufferer from pulmonary trouble than Colorado.[43]

As a result of reports like Iddings's, TB patients flocked to communities in the foothills and mountains of Colorado. Entire towns with inspirational names like Montcalm, Sunny Rest, and Hygiene sprang up around the founding of Sanatoria.[44] Several places became particularly notable (Boulder and Manitou Springs), where guests were treated to spa-like conditions including mineral baths, daily massages, exotic foods, and live music. Likewise, the expansive verandas afforded recovering patients spectacular views of the mountain scenery.

Given its sizeable population, extensive health-care services, and abundant housing options, Denver became a hot spot for treating TB patients. However, because not everyone could afford luxurious mountainside accommodations, local benefactors established hospitals dedicated to treating tuberculosis patients. Denver's National Jewish Hospital, for example, reserved an entire wing for consumptive cases and provided treatment free of cost to the indigent. The generous services attracted even more lungers to the Mile High City. Around the turn of the twentieth century, one-third of Denver's total population was made up of the one-lung army.[45] By the 1920s however, the welcome mat had been removed and TB sufferers were forced (literally in many cases) to look elsewhere.

Around the same time Denver's TB population began to grow, Colorado Springs was transformed from a small town at the foot of Pikes Peak to a thriving city. Colorado Springs's rapid population growth and economic foundation during the late- nineteenth and early-twentieth centuries is directly tied to the city's successful marketing campaign.[46] Beginning with Dr. Edwin Solly in the mid-1870s and reinforced by other leading physicians, local business interests sent advertisements across the country extolling the city's ideal climate for TB sufferers. Colorado Springs's first hospital opened in 1888 with one of its three buildings dedicated to treating tuberculosis patients. A multitude of sanatoria soon followed. By the 1890s, Colorado Springs had become known as "a most desirable destination for consumptives."[47] The culmination of the marketing scheme came in 1899 when *Mountain Sunshine* magazine became an important tool in solidifying the city's reputation as a haven for health seekers.

In 1901, Colorado Springs's most unusual sanatorium began treating patients.[48] Incorporating the latest in TB research and technology, the Nordrach Ranch Sanatorium featured seventy-two well-ventilated, canvas huts (tepee-looking tents) where patients were exposed to fresh, dry, mountain air 24 hours a day, 365 days a year. Around the turn of the twentieth century, there were no fewer than 17 sanatoria in the greater Colorado Springs area caring for tens of thousands of patients.[49] "For more than 50 years after its founding, Colorado Springs flourished on a bedrock of bacteria."[50]

Many places throughout central and western Colorado attributed their existence to TB treatment facilities and restoring people to full health. In 1900, one-third of Colorado residents were living in the state because of tuberculosis. It is remarkable that Colorado attracted more people seeking a cure for tuberculosis than it did during the famous gold and silver rushes.[51] As a result of the volume of lungers and the cutting-edge research, Colorado became known as the World's Sanatorium.[52]

By the end of the nineteenth century, medical personnel had established that tuberculosis was transmitted through sputum and quarantining infected individuals was the most effective strategy for preventing outbreaks. Although climatic conditions may have eased some of the symptoms of consumption, they played a negligible role in the actual cure of the disease. Despite advances in medical knowledge, the construction of new sanatoria continued into the 1920s, with their numbers peaking in the US by the late 1940s. The discovery of antibiotics in 1943 closed the chapter on major TB outbreaks in Europe and the United States. With the widespread availability of streptomycin and isoniazid in the middle of the twentieth century, most sanatoria ceased operations.[53]

Prior to the turn of the twentieth century, communicable diseases claimed countless lives, and health-care professionals urgently sought therapies that would ease symptoms and cure disease. This chapter has identified two pivotal points in US history when nature-based places with distinct natural qualities were used as a tool to treat physical ailments as well as poor mental and emotional health. Specifically, it highlights how geothermal hot springs and high-elevation sanatoria became widely popular tools for healing and personal restoration. Balneotherapy and hydrotherapy emerged as popular treatments for various skin conditions, physical ailments, and muscle tension. Reports frequently extolled the benefits of soaking in mineral-rich hot springs, asserting that individuals who arrived frail often left restored to full health. Similarly, isolating tuberculosis patients in sanatoria, particularly in high-elevation locations with warm, dry air, was regarded as a particularly effective therapy. Between 1880 and 1920, the American West (most notably Colorado Springs and southern Arizona) became the preferred destination for those seeking recovery from TB. However, following World War II, the number of individuals visiting hot springs for medicinal purposes declined sharply. With the advent of streptomycin, the need for tuberculosis sanatoria vanished. By the late 1970s, most sanatoria had closed or were converted to other uses. Similarly, the once-thriving bathhouses of Hot Springs, Arkansas fell into disuse. The row of once-majestic spas was relegated to a landmark on the National Historic Registry and transformed into a tourist attraction.

Today, although we recognize that hot springs and sanatoria were not the cure-alls people once thought, they nevertheless retain an enduring legacy as sites of healing and renewal. Even though their medical efficacy proved limited, these places were widely perceived as havens of restoration and personal well-being. Soaking in geothermal waters remains a deeply soothing and rejuvenating experience, and the cultural significance of hot springs and health spas endures across the globe. From Middle Eastern hammams and Eastern European banyas to Iceland's geyser-fed hot pools and Japanese onsens, hydrothermal bathing persist as integral components of wellness practices. In recent years, luxury health spas and wellness centers have experienced a remarkable resurgence, offering exclusive, cutting-edge treatments designed to promote holistic restoration.[54] Many of these elite facilities are located in remote, idyllic locations and cater to individuals of considerable financial means. And yet, the restorative potential of nature is not restricted to these exclusive therapeutic destinations. Nature remains accessible to people of all backgrounds and is as near as the closest park, forest, or natural recreation area. Nature continues to serve as a vital sanctuary for personal restoration.

Conclusion

Lessons from the Past, Insights for the Future

For most of human history, people lived in rural areas because their livelihoods were directly tied to the land. Before the Industrial Revolution, work was physically demanding, and daily life involved regular exposure to nature. Since industrialization, however, people have gravitated toward cities. In the US, the urban population grew from 51 percent in 1920 to more than 80 percent today.

As people flock to cities, they tend to become more detached from nature.[1] In OECD countries (including the US) individuals now spend most of their time indoors. A recent study found that more than half (51 percent) of Americans spend less than three times per month in nature, with 16 percent of US residents spending no time interacting with nature at all.[2] Furthermore, researchers at the Harvard School of Public Health found that Americans spend more time in their vehicles than outdoors.[3] This shift has raised concerns among health professionals because, as people spend more time gazing at screens than being outside, they miss the health benefits that nature offers.[4]

With the rise of sedentary and urban lifestyles, mental health issues like stress, anxiety, and depression have become more prevalent.[5] Health journalist Richard Louv refers to this syndrome as "nature-deficit disorder," linking it to shorter attention spans and higher rates of physical and emotional distress.[6] Depression rates among US adults have increased from 5.4 percent in 2005 to 18 percent in 2023.[7] Oxford University Press named "brain rot" the 2024 word of the year, a term that captures the perceived adverse effects of excessive social media and smartphone use on mental health.[8]

In 2025, Douglas Harris and his colleagues released their *State of the Nation* report, assessing overall quality of life in the US. Built around thirty-seven variables, including the economy, education, employment, environment, individual health, national security, and violence, the report found that US mental health is in severe decline. Moreover, the United States ranks near the bottom among 114 countries examined; only 13 countries report worse mental health.[9]

Poor mental health stems from various factors, including genetic, sociocultural (age, gender, income, occupation, relationships), and environmental (abuse, conflict, isolation, trauma, violence). However, research increasingly points to sensory overload as a leading risk factor.[10] This occurs when one or more senses are overstimulated by the immediate environment. Many characteristics associated with urbanization (noise, congestion, pollution) are key triggers. People living in highly urbanized areas are now ten times more likely to suffer from mental health disorders (especially anxiety and depression) than they were sixty years ago.[11] Renewal and restoration can come in many forms (listening to music, reading, shopping, exercising), but research shows it is most effective when individuals have a place where they can retreat (escape) from the mental and emotional stress associated with modern, urban living.[12]

In the early 1990s, scholars began linking specific places with favorable health outcomes, recognizing that some environments appear to have healing properties. Drawing upon his scholastic background in humanistic geography and the geographies of health, Wilbert Gesler coined the term "therapeutic landscape."[13] Research soon expanded to include sites with long-established healing reputations (spa towns), landscapes of considerable natural beauty (mountainous and seaside locations), and spiritual retreats (sacred sites).[14] By the early 2000s, therapeutic landscapes had become a recognized field of study.

Alongside research on therapeutic landscapes, environmental psychologists have studied how certain environments influence health and well-being. First introduced by Stephen and Rachel Kaplan, "restorative environments" are settings that help reduce stress, calm the mind, and engage the senses.[15] Two theories emerged (Psycho-Evolutionary Theory and Attention Restoration Theory). Both assert that restorative places allow the brain to disengage, enable individuals to effortlessly absorb the qualities of their surroundings, and afford the brain time to restore its capacity to function properly.[16]

Both therapeutic landscapes and restorative environments focus on human-environment interaction, but they differ in their methods. Scholars of therapeutic landscapes typically take a humanistic, qualitative approach[17] and have recently explored social networking and the symbolic meaning of places.[18] By comparison, environmental psychologists tend to use quantitative methods to measure emotional and physical restoration associated with particular places.[19] Despite methodological differences, both fields aim to understand the social, material, and emotional qualities inherent in places that promote healing and personal well-being.[20]

In 1984, Roger Ulrich was the first scholar to explore the connection between people's interaction with nature and personal health. Ulrich found that patients assigned to rooms with a view of a natural setting recovered faster and required fewer analgesics than those facing a brick wall.[21] Since then, environmental psychologists, social epidemiologists, and landscape architects have led a growing body of research on the health benefits of interacting with nature[22] (Table 6.1). As Terry Hartig notes, "People have a biologically prepared capacity for acquiring and retaining restorative responses to certain nature settings . . . but have no such disposition for most built environments."[23]

Despite significant progress in understanding therapeutic landscapes and restorative environments, little scholarship has explored the historical roots of today's restorative places. Our understanding of where and how these places originated remains incomplete. This book addresses that gap in the literature by providing a historical and geographical account of how nature has been used as a tool to combat physical, cognitive, and emotional illness. It examines pivotal milestones and sociocultural forces that have shaped the role of nature-based places in human restoration. This concluding chapter highlights lessons learned from this perspective that remain relevant today. It helps address such questions as: What were the origins of restorative places? What sites first served as retreats from the challenges of modern urban living? What societal and technological changes spurred the rise of restorative places for the masses? How have the unique qualities of nature-based places supported healing over time? Where have city dwellers historically found refuge within their own communities? Ultimately, this book reinforces the theoretical foundations of restorative environments (especially Psycho-Evolutionary Theory and Attention Restoration Theory) by

Table 6.1. Health Benefits of Routine Positive Interaction with Nature

Physical Benefits	Mental/Emotional Benefits
Reduces risk of all-cause mortality	Improves cognition and brain health
Lowers risk of heart disease and stroke	Reduces risk of depression
Improves metabolic health	Reduces feelings of anxiety
Improves cardiovascular functions	Reduces stress and rumination
Reduces hypertension	Reduces cortisol levels
Lowers risk of Type 2 diabetes	Boosts endorphin levels
Improves blood lipid profile	Improves dopamine and serotonin levels
Lowers risk of some cancers	Reduces postpartum depression
Improves respiratory capacity	Reduces Seasonal Affective Disorder
Reduces risk of obesity	Reduces risk of dementia/Alzheimer's
Improves weight management	Increases attention and focus
Improves gastrointestinal function	Improves crystallized and fluid
Improves bone health	Improves mental processing speed
Improves joint health & physical function	Reduces symptoms of ADHD in children
Improves muscle fitness	Boosts creative thinking
Improves quality of sleep	Provides free aromatherapy
Improves overall physical fitness	Reduces risk of falls in older adults
Reduces inflammation & physical discomfort	
Improves renal functions	
Boosts immune system	
Boosts energy levels	
Improves appetite	
Improves vision	
Boosts Vitamin D intake	
Improves gestation	

Sources: APA 2020; Bratman *et al.* 2015; CDC 2022; Hartig *et al.* 2014; Kaplan 1995; Maller *et al.* 2005; Piercy *et al.* 2018; Scopelliti *et al.* 2019; Takano *et al.* 2002; Ulrich 1984.

illustrating how certain places have long provided recreation, refuge, and retreat from the stresses of modern urban life. The overall takeaway is that, although sociocultural forces and technology continue to change, nature's role as a source of personal restoration remains constant, a principle now recognized as "cultural ecosystem services."[24]

Origins

At the turn of the nineteenth century, US government officials and corporate executives viewed nature as an obstacle to progress, something that needed to be tamed and conquered. However, some of the nation's most influential philosophers and writers saw nature differently. They held grave concerns about the harmful effects of urban living and the reckless destruction of wilderness. Two of nature's most ardent advocates were Henry David Thoreau and John Muir. As a leading voice of the Transcendentalist Movement, Thoreau railed against the dehumanizing aspects of industrialization and the blatant misery caused by rampant urbanization. He believed city life took a heavy toll, forcing men to lead lives of quiet desperation. Thoreau saw nature as a tonic for the damaged human spirit, offering an ideal setting for personal restoration. Having witnessed firsthand the wanton destruction of nature's beauty, John Muir held a similar sentiment. In his mind, the unbridled pace of urban growth was the greatest threat to nature. His passion for wilderness preservation led him to write, "wilderness is a necessity of life, . . . mountain parks and reservations are useful not only as fountains of timber and irrigating rivers, but as fountains of life."[25] Both Thoreau and Muir sought to change how Americans viewed nature, emphasizing its vital role in healing and personal well-being.

In this cultural climate, the Hudson River School of landscape painting emerged. As the nation's first major art movement, it gave visual expression to transcendentalist ideals and further shaped public perceptions of wilderness. Early painters like Thomas Cole and Asher B. Durand depicted nature's divine and sublime qualities, while later artists sought to capture the restorative qualities of nature. Albert Bierstadt's prolific, vivid, and lifelike paintings of the mountainous West inspired awe and imagination transporting viewers to a world far removed from the stresses and strains of everyday urban living. His "Great Pictures" exhibitions drew large crowds eager to find moments of peace, solace, and contentment in the beauty of nature. Consistent with Terry Hartig's research, the Hudson River School's paintings are among the earliest examples of nature being used as a tool for personal restoration. By offering an escape from stress and anxiety while engaging viewers in fascination, they highlight nature's psychological benefits, an effect that remains relevant today.

First Retreats

In the late 1800s and early 1900s, affluent households had little trouble escaping the stresses of urban life, thanks to ample time, money, and improved transportation. Steamships and railroads opened new travel opportunities, allowing America's elite to venture beyond East Coast city limits. Early on, the Catskills and Poconos became popular retreats for well-to-do households, yet exploring deep into the untamed wilds of nature remained uncommon. That changed in 1869, when William H. H. Murray's book inspired wealthy urbanites to explore the Adirondack Mountains of upstate New York. The Congregational minister's work highlighted the health-giving and spirit-enhancing benefits of communing with nature. Enthralled by his message, well-heeled urbanites flocked to the Adirondacks. Initially, wealthy families camped in tents or rented simple cabins, but over time, the rustic lodging gave way to lavish resorts. Some of the most prominent families even built private summer retreats, known as "great camps."

The fresh mountain air provided a peaceful escape, allowing them to recharge their mental and physical capacities. As middle-class families began discovering these scenic uplands, the elite shifted their attention to the White Mountains of northern New Hampshire and Maine. Crawford Path emerged as the nation's first hiking trail designed for outdoor recreation, with many hiring guides for climbs up Mount Washington. Over time, the affluent urbanites formed hiking and adventure clubs and blazed a vast network of hiking paths along the Atlantic Seaboard. This growing enthusiasm inspired Benton MacKaye to propose a single continuous trail through the East Coast uplands.[26] Completed in 1937, the Appalachian Trail solidified these mountains as centers of personal restoration. In succession, the Catskills, Poconos, Adirondacks, and White Mountains became the earliest retreats from the stresses of modern urban living.

Societal and Technological Changes

Following the American Civil War, the Gilded Age witnessed significant economic growth alongside widespread worker exploitation. After Theodore Roosevelt's inauguration, the nation made strides in labor reform. Spearheaded by the Ford Motor Company, the standard workweek was reduced from sixty to forty hours, granting laborers not only improved working conditions but also more leisure time for rest and rejuvenation. As reform efforts took hold, more households gained access to the healing benefits of nature. Yet, despite having more leisure time, many households still struggled to escape to nature due to the high cost of train and steamship tickets. The advent of mass-produced automobiles changed that. As Ford's affordable cars became readily available, middle-class families could easily escape urban centers. Sunday drives in the country became a popular remedy for urban fatigue.

Many destinations capitalized on this newfound mobility afforded by private automobiles. For example, Point Lobos on the western edge of San Francisco Peninsula became a haven for nature lovers and those seeking relief from the ills of city life. In the Rocky Mountain West, Denver, Colorado pioneered the concept of a mountain park system, later expanded through Jefferson County Open Space. Aimed at enhancing community health, Denver metropolitan area governments have worked to preserve natural areas where both residents and visitors can escape urban pressures and connect with nature. These experiences became widely accessible thanks to labor reform and the advent of affordable private transportation.

Today, scenic drives remain a cherished way to experience nature. In Denver, the Lariat Loop and the breathtaking road up Mount Evans (now called Mount Blue Sky) continue to offer escapes into the mountains. Across the country, scenic byways like the Pacific Coast Highway, Blue Ridge Parkway, and Trail of the Ancients provide similar experiences. One of the most striking is Colorado's Alpine Loop, a rugged off-highway vehicle (OHV) route through the San Juan Mountains, linking the towns of Ouray, Lake City, and Silverton (Figure 6.1). Much like the Lariat Loop a century ago, this drive offers a retreat from urban life, featuring views of towering peaks, ghost towns, and abandoned mining camps. Aligned with Psycho-Evolutionary Theory (PET) and Attention Restoration Theory (ART), the Alpine Loop embodies two key elements of restorative places, being away and fascination.[27]

Unique Qualities of Place

At the turn of the twentieth century, infectious diseases like pneumonia and tuberculosis were the leading causes of death. In their search for alternative therapies, doctors looked for places with unique natural qualities believed to promote healing. Among the many therapeutic landscapes identified in the US, two locations gained prominence for their perceived restorative benefits. These places possessed distinct natural elements believed to support healing, renewal, and personal well-being.

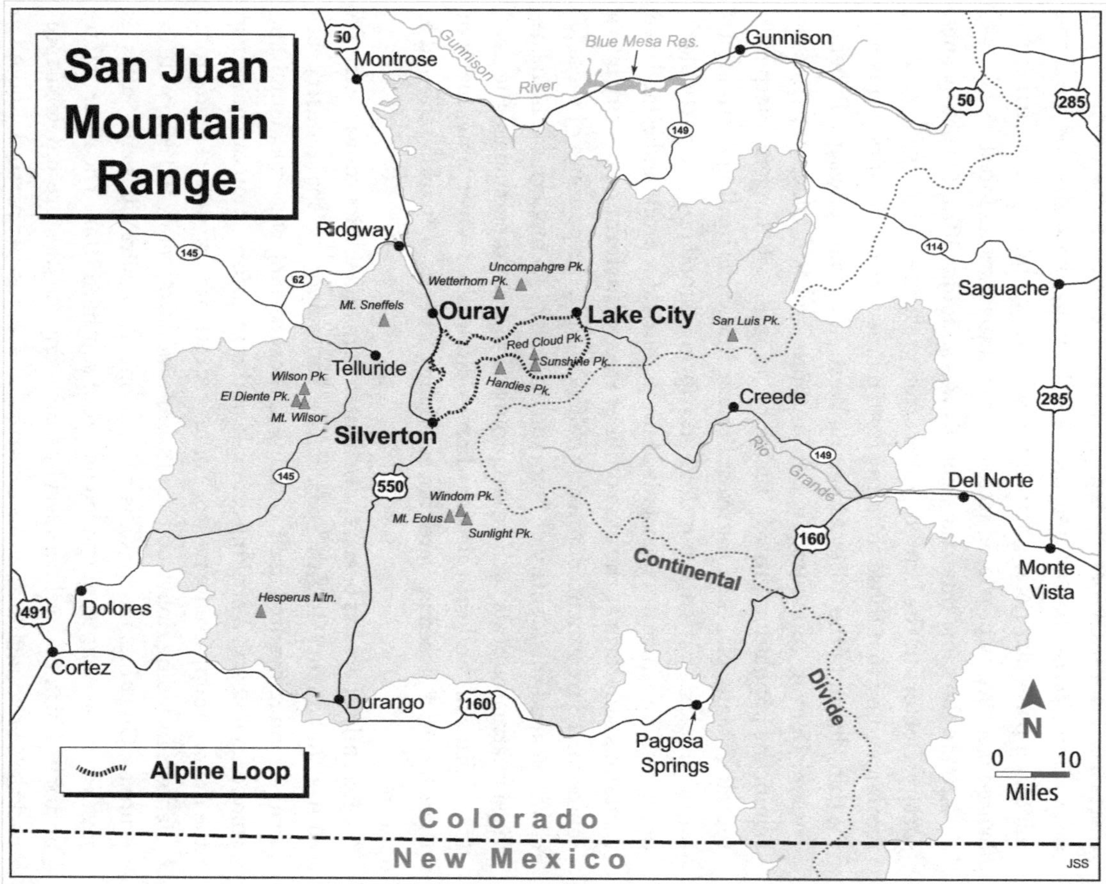

Figure 6.1 Map of San Juan Mountains and Alpine Loop. Cartography by Jeffrey S. Smith.

In 1832, the US government designated Hot Springs, Arkansas, as a Federal Reservation and fifty years later it established the country's first health spa. By the early 1900s, people with various ailments found their way to the Ouachita Mountains of west-central Arkansas to soak in the area's geothermal bathhouses. What started as a cure for physical diseases evolved into a restorative place that treated people holistically (both the body and the mind). Of particular note, a network of color-coded hiking trails further enhanced recovery by providing access to the nearby tranquil forest.

Around the same time, tuberculosis was a raging infirmity that plagued society. Doctors in the United States often prescribed a change in climate, recommending that those suffering from pulmonary consumption travel to the thin, dry air of the Rocky Mountain West. As a result, cities like Phoenix, Tucson, Denver, Albuquerque, San Antonio, and San Diego experienced significant population growth, fueled by an influx of "lungers," desperate for relief. Many places in the West became known as healing destinations for tuberculosis patients, but Colorado Springs stood out as a particularly prominent hub. Investors recognized the potential for profit and established numerous sanatoria at the base of Pikes Peak, transforming the city into a center for TB treatment. For nearly half a century, the presence of these facilities shaped the identity of Colorado Springs.[28] As modern medicine devised pharmaceuticals such as streptomycin to treat tuberculosis, the need for health spas and convalescent homes diminished. Over time, many of these facilities closed or were converted into other uses, marking the end of an era.

Recently, there has been renewed interest in full-service convalescent facilities and luxury health spas.[29] The contemporary spa industry has adapted and reinvented itself, catering to those seeking physical, mental, and emotional renewal. A striking example of this transformation can be seen in the Aman Group, an elite network of luxury retreats that attract high-profile clientele, including Hollywood actors, professional athletes, and corporate executives. One of its most exclusive locations (Amangiri Villas and Suites) is nestled in the remote, unspoiled desert of southern Utah. The resort offers an array of high-end wellness services, including the "Restore and Rebalance" package (a two-night experience starting at $10,000 per person). Rooted in traditional Navajo *hózhó* healing practices, this program integrates the elements of earth, wind, fire, and water to restore harmony and balance. Guests receive a personalized wellness consultation, spa treatments, massages, and a Crystal Sound Bath, along with access to more than thirty outdoor activities, such as horseback riding, nature hikes, cable walks, and guided canyon tours. For an additional $8,500, guests can take a helicopter to Tower Butte for a sunrise yoga session led by a master instructor. According to the Amangiri website, these carefully crafted experiences are designed to provide "a balm for the restlessness brought on by the frenetic pace of modern life," allowing guests to "leave feeling restored and rejuvenated."[30] Although the setting and clientele may differ from the bathhouses and tuberculosis sanatoria of the past, the underlying philosophy remains remarkably similar, offering a retreat where nature, fresh air, and physical activity are central to the healing process. Many of today's most sought-after wellness centers are, in essence, modern adaptations of age-old therapeutic traditions that have long emphasized the restorative power of nature.

Refuge Within Cities

As awareness of nature's healing qualities grew, visionary leaders sought ways to make urban life more desirable and restorative. William Cullen Bryant, for example, championed city parks, believing that those who have become burdened by the "sorrows, crimes, and incivility of cities" should have the opportunity to "enter the woods and view the haunts of nature" to find peace and serenity.[31] In 1858, Frederick Law Olmsted and Calvert Vaux's vision for Central Park not only established a restorative place within New York City's urban fabric, but also laid the groundwork for the City Beautiful Movement. Chicago's World's Fair and Washington DC's National Mall demonstrated how cities could be both functional and restorative. In the ensuing decades, many midsized cities, such as Birmingham, Buffalo, Denver, and Milwaukee, followed their lead. With its tree-lined boulevards, fountains, scenic parkways, and abundant public parks, no city embraced the City Beautiful Movement more fully than Kansas City, Missouri, investments that continue to pay dividends today. By the 1990s landscape architects and city planners embraced a new urban paradigm known as restorative environmental design (RED). Building on biophilic design (which integrates nature into the built environment), RED seeks to foster connections to nature by prioritizing urban spaces that nurture both physical and psychological well-being.[32] By the mid-2000s, cities across the country had set aside sizable parklands and developed networks of hiking trails. Major urban centers like Atlanta, Baltimore, Boston, Chicago, and Philadelphia introduced pocket parks and small public urban green spaces (SPUGs), while cities such as Phoenix and San Antonio utilized riparian zones for water management and outdoor recreation.[33] Many cities nationwide have integrated green space into their urban fabric, but none has surpassed Portland, Oregon, in setting aside restorative spaces for its residents.[34] With more than 200 community parks, 250,000 trees, and 150 miles of hiking trails, its award-winning Parks and Recreation Department has shaped the city into a sanctuary for nature lovers. By prioritizing access to nature, Portland has successfully realized its vision of enhancing mental and physical health through outdoor recreation.[35]

Spectrum of Nature-Based Experiences and Barriers to Access

The case studies presented in this book illustrate that nature-based experiences exist on a continuum, ranging from indirect encounters like viewing landscape paintings to direct activities such as driving in the mountains or hiking through a forest. To fully benefit from nature's healing, rejuvenating, and restorative qualities, individuals must choose experiences that align with their comfort levels, cultural traditions, and physical abilities. Simply put, an outdoor experience must be accessible and personally fulfilling if it is to serve as an escape from the stresses of urban living.

Despite the well-documented benefits of spending time in nature, participation rates vary significantly. A recent survey found that 53 percent of American adults regularly engage in outdoor activities (excluding organized sports), while one-third (31 percent) participate infrequently (less than once a month) or not at all[36] (Table 6.2). The reasons for this disparity are complex. Nearly 45 percent of individuals cite time constraints (demanding jobs, busy schedules, and family obligations) as the primary barrier to outdoor engagement (Table 6.3). Furthermore, the health benefits of interacting with nature do not seem to accrue to all segments of society. Although 72 percent of White (non-Hispanic) Americans participate in nature-based activities on a regular basis, only 12 percent of Latinx/Hispanic individuals and 9 percent of Black (African American) do so (Table 6.4). These disparities point to larger sociocultural and systemic issues, including economic barriers, historical exclusion from outdoor spaces, and differences in how various communities engage with nature. To address these inequities, various government agencies have implemented initiatives aimed at increasing outdoor participation

Table 6.2. Participation in Nature-Based Outdoor Recreation, 2020

Frequency	Percent of Population Participating
Overall participation rate 52.9%	
Multiple times each week	26%
Once a week	22%
Once or twice per month	20%
Less than once a month	15%
Never	16%
Total US Population (331 million)	

Sources: OF 2021; US Bureau of the Census, 2021.

Table 6.3. Reasons Given for Not Interacting with Nature, 2020

Reason Given	Percent of Respondents
Job demands too much time	31%
Health issues/disability	9%
General lack of time/too busy	7%
Family, school, or other obligations	5%
Weather	4%
No interest/do other things	3%
Can't afford doing it	2%
Outdoor hazards (bugs, pollen, sun)	2%
Too old/age	2%
Transportation logistics	2%
Other	5%

Sources: Adapted from Quinn and Helmstetter 2019.
Data from APM Survey.

among underrepresented groups.[37] The US National Park Service, for example, has prioritized efforts to attract a more diverse population to national parks and monuments.[38] For these programs to be successful, more research is needed to better understand the cultural, economic, and logistical barriers that limit outdoor participation.

Physical ability is another significant obstacle to nature engagement. The second most common reason cited for not participating in outdoor activities

Table 6.4. Adult Participation in Nature-Based Outdoor Recreation by Demographic Group, 2020

Demographic Group	Percent of Total US Population	Percent of Total Participating
Overall participation 160.7 million (52.9%)		
Females	50.5%	46.2%
Males	49.5%	53.8%
White (non-Hispanic)	60.9%	71.5%
Hispanic/Latinx	17.9%	11.6%
African-American	12.4%	9.4%
Asian-American	5.8%	6.0%
Total US Population (2020): 331 million		

Sources: OF 2021; US Bureau of the Census.

is health issues or disability[39] (Table 6.3). A major criticism of the growing EcoWellness Movement is that its benefits disproportionately serve able-bodied individuals, often overlooking the needs of individuals with physical disabilities.[40] Despite increasing awareness of accessibility issues, many outdoor spaces remain difficult for individuals with mobility impairments to navigate. For example, although the Denver Mountain Park system and Jefferson County Open Space (JCOS) parks have been widely celebrated for their scenic beauty and preservation of green space, one of the most frequent complaints is their lack of ADA-compliant trails and facilities.[41] The Americans with Disabilities Act of 1990 mandates that city parks within urban areas be accessible, but these regulations rarely extend to peri-urban and exurban parks, leaving many natural areas out of reach for those with mobility challenges. Improving accessibility is an intuitive and necessary step in ensuring that nature remains a restorative space for all individuals, regardless of physical ability.

One initiative that has successfully addressed this gap is Wilderness on Wheels. Located about 60 miles west of Denver along US Highway 285 (Figure 3.5), the facility opened in 1986 after taking fifteen years to construct. The 20-acre site features two boardwalk paths, picnic tables, campsites, cabins, and a fishing pond.[42] The pinnacle activity is a strenuous, mile-long climb to an elevation of 9,000 feet. At the top, an overlook offers panoramic views of the valley below. Open from Memorial Day

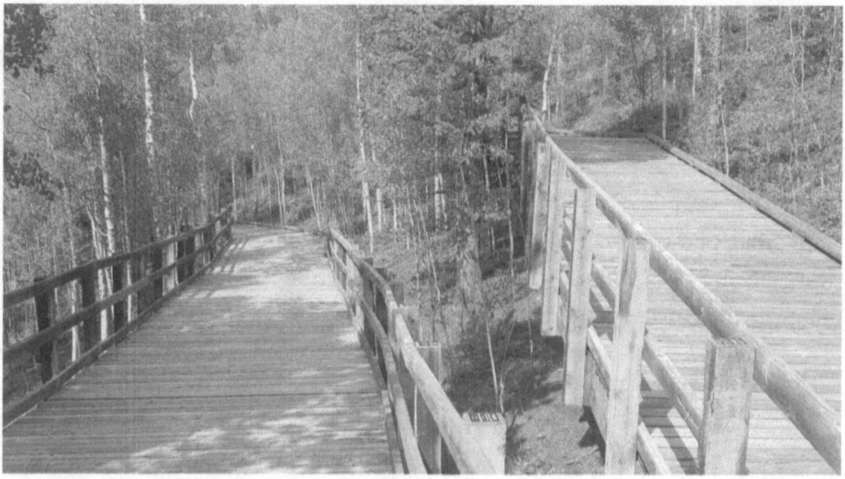

Figure 6.2 Photo of Boardwalk Through Nature at Wilderness on Wheels. Photo by Jeffrey S. Smith, 2021.

through mid-October, Wilderness on Wheels provides individuals of all abilities the opportunity to immerse themselves in nature, listen to the sound of aspen trees quaking in the breeze, and find solace in a wilderness setting (Figure 6.2). Places like Wilderness on Wheels illustrate the importance of creating restorative environments that accommodate diverse populations. They also align with theories such as Psycho-Evolutionary Theory (PET) and Attention Restoration Theory (ART), which emphasize the restorative effects of nature and its ability to captivate attention in a way that promotes rejuvenation and personal well-being. However, more research is needed to explore what restorative places look like for different demographic groups, including the elderly, people of color, and individuals with disabilities. These discussions also intersect with broader themes of accessibility, modernization, and democratization, which have historically shaped (and continue to influence) who interacts with nature.

The Democratization of Restorative Places

Historically, access to nature was largely stratified by class. In the nineteenth century, the ability to retreat into nature was a privilege of the wealthy. They had both the leisure time and financial means to escape city life and explore remote lands. Exclusive mountain resorts catered to the rich and famous, providing sanctuaries for rest and restoration. In many ways, the idea of nature as a healthful refuge was shaped by these early elite experiences and reinforced the idea that immersion in scenic landscapes promoted physical and mental well-being. Changes in society, however, gradually broadened access to restorative places. The labor reform movement granted laborers shorter work hours and weekends off, providing working- and middle-class Americans with increased leisure time. This allowed them to engage with nature in ways previously reserved for elites. These changes were further accelerated by improvements in transportation technology.

In the mid- to late-nineteenth century, the rise of steamships and railroads enabled greater access to nature. The Poconos, Catskills, and Adirondacks all gained in popularity because the new modes of transportation replaced what had previously been accessible only by horse and carriage. This era also witnessed the expansion of the sanatorium movement, due in part to the completion of the southern transcontinental railroad. Tuberculosis patients headed west to California, Arizona, and Colorado in search of dry, healing climates. Meanwhile, the urban parks movement (exemplified by Frederick Law Olmsted's design of Central Park) created restorative green spaces within industrializing cities, thereby providing access to nature for those who could not afford out-of-town travel.

By the early twentieth century, the widespread adoption of private automobiles further transformed the geography of therapeutic landscapes. Cars enabled middle- and working-class households to embark on nature excursions, fueling the rise of roadside motels, campgrounds, and auto-touring culture. National parks like Yellowstone and Yosemite (once the domain of elite rail-based tourism) became more accessible to the general public. The development of scenic highways and mountain park systems reinforced the idea that nature should be available to all, not just the privileged few. As transportation and labor conditions improved, access to nature became increasingly democratized.

The historical trajectory of restorative places (from exclusive retreats to public parks to the automobile-driven expansion of outdoor recreation) offers valuable lessons for the present. Long before cultural ecosystem services became a defined research topic, the case studies explored in this book illustrate the deep, intangible benefits that nature has provided (including recreation, inspiration, and personal renewal) across different eras. In whatever form it has taken, interacting with nature has long been valued not only for its physical health benefits but also for the ways it enriches human experience.

Today, while many historical barriers to nature have been addressed, new challenges are emerging, especially as modern society contends with the rise of digital technology. What will the future of restorative places look like? Emerging trends suggest a growing emphasis on digital detox retreats (a movement that acknowledges both the benefits of nature and the need to disconnect from an increasingly technology-saturated world). Concepts like "second life" and virtual restorative environments (including online meditation spaces and Immersive Virtual Reality experiences) hint at a potential shift in how individuals seek nature-based restoration. While these technological advancements could offer new ways to engage with nature, they also raise critical questions about authenticity, accessibility, and the evolving relationship between humans and the natural world.

A Lasting Bond with Place

Finally, restorative places are more than just physical locations or abstract natural settings devoid of meaning. As individuals return to these spaces time and again, they develop a profound connection (i.e., place attachment) to them (one that shapes their identity and sense of well-being).[43] These places become more than just settings of recovery and rejuvenation; they become integral to a person's life story, fostering a deep sense of belonging.

Recent scholarship identifies six types of places to which people form emotional attachments.[44] Among them, transformative places are especially noteworthy. These are sites where profound, life-altering experiences occur. In such places, individuals often emerge with a renewed sense of energy and vitality, restored from periods of stress, environmental fatigue, or personal challenges. Consequently, restorative places serve as catalysts for transformation, becoming inseparable from the journey toward personal well-being. The emotional attachment people develop toward such places stems from the significant transformations experienced in that location.

These attachments extend beyond the individual. Whether through personal experiences, generational traditions (such as a family hike or an annual retreat), or shared community practices (like public gatherings in a neighborhood green space), restorative places become part of the collective consciousness. The bonds people form with these landscapes influence how they perceive, engage with, and care for the environment, fostering a collective sense of responsibility for its care and preservation.

At the community level, people rally around places that define them, advocating for their preservation. They push for policies that protect open space and work to ensure that future generations can experience the same sense of peace, comfort, and renewal. These efforts speak to an essential truth: restorative places are not just valuable; they are vital. As society continues to evolve, ensuring that these places remain protected and accessible will be essential to the well-being of individuals and communities alike.

Notes

Introduction

1. Twain (1864), *A Trip to the Cliff House*.

2. Cutler (2009), *Sutro Baths*; Delgado *et al.* (2000), *The History and Significance of the Adolph Sutro Historic District*.

3. Delgado *et al.* (2000), *The History and Significance of the Adolph Sutro Historic District*.

4. Smith (2005), *San Francisco's Lost Landmarks*.

5. Nemade and Patricelli (2020), *Historical Understanding of Depression*.

6. Khodaei *et al.* (2017), *Avicenna (980–1032 CE)*.

7. Schimelpfening and Morin (2020), *The History of Depression*.

8. Ilardi (2009), *The Depression Cure*.

9. Anderson *et al.* (2017), *Lively Social Space, Well-Being Activity, and Urban Design*; Clancy and Ryan (2015), *The Role of Biophilic Design in Landscape Architecture for Health and Well-Being*; Kaplan (1995), *The Restorative Benefits of Nature*; Maller *et al.* (2009), *Rediscovering Nature in Everyday Settings*.

10. MacKerron and Mourato (2013), *Happiness is Greater in Natural Environments*.

11. Berto (2014), *The Role of Nature in Coping with Psycho-Physiological Stress*.

12. Kaplan and Kaplan (1989), *The Experience of Nature*.

13. Hug *et al.* (2009), *Restorative Qualities of Indoor and Outdoor Exercise Settings as Predictors of Exercise Frequency*; Rosenbaum and Wong (2015), *The Restorative Potential of Casinos*; Rosenbaum *et al.* (2016), *The Restorative Potential of Shopping Malls*.

14. Brewster (2014), *The Public Library as Therapeutic Landscape*; Packer and Bond (2010), *Museums as Restorative Environments*.

15. Berto (2014), *The Role of Nature in Coping with Psycho-Physiological Stress*; Herzog *et al.* (2003), *Assessing the Restorative Components of Environments*; Kaplan (1995), *The Restorative Benefits of Nature*; Schebella *et al.* (2017), *For the Love of Nature*; Scopelliti *et al.* (2019), *Is it Really Nature that Restores People?*; Subiza-Perez *et al.* (2020), *Welcome to Your Plaza*.

16. Jett (1992), *An Introduction of Navajo Sacred Place*, 30.

17. Blake (2001), *Contested Landscapes of Navajo Sacred Mountains;* Kahn-John and Koithan (2015), *Living in Health, Harmony, and Beauty*.

18. Hartig (2011), *Issues in Restorative Environments Research*.

19. Bell *et al.* (2017), *Using Geonarratives to Explore the Diverse Temporalities of Therapeutic Landscapes*; Bell, *et al.* (2018), *From Therapeutic Landscapes to Healthy Spaces, Places and Practices*; Collins (2020), *The Architecture and Landscape of Health*; Gesler (2003), *Healing Places*; Glass and Singer (1972), *Urban Stress*; Laws (2009), *Reworking Therapeutic*

Landscapes; Williams (1999), *Therapeutic Landscapes*; Wohlwill (1974), *Human Adaptation to Levels of Environmental Stimulation*.

20. Hartig (2011), *Issues in Restorative Environments Research*; Negrin *et al.* (2017), *Discrimination of Urban Spaces with Different Level of Restorativeness Based on the Original and on a Shorter Version of Hartig et al.'s Perceived Restorativeness Scale*.

21. Hartig *et al.* (1997), *A Measure of Restorative Qualities in Environments*; Kaplan and Kaplan (1989), *The Experience of Nature*.

22. Hartig (2011), *Issues in Restorative Environments Research*; Kaplan (1995), *The Restorative Benefits of Nature*; Scopelliti and Giuliani (2004), *Choosing Restorative Environments Across the Lifespan*.

23. Fornara and Troffa (2009), *Restorative Experiences and Perceived Affective Qualities in Different Built and Natural Urban Places*; Lehto (2012), *Assessing the Perceived Restorative Qualities of Vacation Destinations;* Subiza-Perez *et al.* (2020), *Welcome to Your Plaza*.

24. Bodin and Hartig (2003), *Does the Outdoor Environment Matter for Psychological Restoration Gained Through Running?*; Hartig and Staats (2006), *The Need for Psychological Restoration as a Determinant of Environmental Preferences*.

25. Herzog *et al.* (2003), *Assessing the Restorative Components of Environments*; Korpela *et al.* (2008), *Determinants of Restorative Experiences in Everyday Favorite Places*; Nordh, *et al.* (2009), *Components of Small Urban Parks that Predict the Possibility of Restoration*.

26. Hansmann *et al.* (2007), *Restoration and Stress Relief Through Physical Activities in Forests and Parks*; Hartig *et al.* (2003), *Residence in the Social Ecology of Stress and Restoration*; Staats, *et al.* (2003), *When to Recover from Attentional Fatigue*.

27. For additional information see: Bagot *et al.* (2007), *Amendments to the Perceived Restorative Components Scale for Children*; Berto (2005), *Exposure to Restorative Environments Helps Restore Attentional Capacity*; Carrus *et al.* (2017), *A Different Way to Stay in Touch with 'Urban Nature'*; Gifford (1987), *The Motivation of Park Users*; Han (2003), *A Reliable and Valid Self-Rating Measure of the Restorative Quality of Natural Environments*; Laumann *et al.* (2001), *Rating Scale Measures of Restorative Components of Environments*; Laumann *et al.* (2003), *Selective Attention and Heart Rate Responses to Natural and Urban Environments*; Pals *et al.* (2009), *Development of the PRCQ*; Ulrich (1984), *View Through a Window May Influence Recovery from Surgery*; Van den Berg *et al.* (2014), *Evaluating Restoration in Urban Green Spaces*.

28. Hartig *et al.* (1997), *A Measure of Restorative Qualities in Environments*.

29. Korpela and Hartig (1996), *Restorative Qualities of Favorite Places*; Korpela *et al.* (2001), *Restorative Experience and Self-Regulation in Favorite Places*.

30. Hartig *et al.* (1997), *A Measure of Restorative Qualities in Environments*; Mattila *et al.* (2020), *Restoration in a Virtual Reality Forest Environment*.

31. Browning and Ryan (2020), *Nature Inside*, 2.

32. Wyckoff and Dilsaver (1995), *The Mountainous West*, 4.

33. Buttimer (1976), *Grasping the Dynamism of Lifeworld*; Seamon and Lundberg (2017), *Humanistic Geography*.

34. Jackson (1994), *A Sense of Place, A Sense of Time*.

35. Buttimer and Seamon (1980), *The Human Experience of Space and Place*; Seamon and Lundberg (2017), *Humanistic Geography*; Tuan (1974), *Topophilia*; Tuan (1977), *Space and Place*.

36. Gesler (1992), *Therapeutic Landscapes*.

37. Williams (2009), *Therapeutic Landscapes as Health Promoting Places*.

38. Jensen and Guthrie (2006), *Outdoor Recreation in America*, 41.

39. Harner (2021), *Profiting from the Peak*.

40. NAMI (2020), *Mental Health by the Numbers*.

Chapter 1. Roots of Restoration

1. Kemmis (1990), *Community and the Politics of Place*; Myerson (2000), *Transcendentalism*; Peterson (1991), *Telling the Farmers' Story*.

2. Emerson (1836), *Nature*, 12–14.

3. Schlett (2015), *A Not Too Greatly Changed Eden*.

4. Gura (2007), *American Transcendentalism*; Packer (2007), *The Transcendentalists*.

5. Buell (2003), *Emerson*; Sacks (2003), *Understanding Emerson*.

6. Thoreau (1854), *Walden*.

7. Buell (1995), *The Environmental Imagination*; Curtis (2010), *The Virtue of Thoreau*; Stewart (1995), *A Natural History of Nature Writing*; Walls (2017), *Henry David Thoreau*.

8. Fuller (1845), *Woman in the Nineteenth Century*.

9. Ruskin (1903), *Modern Painters Volume II*.

10. Young (2017), *Heading Out*.

11. Blewitt (2019), *William Morris & John Ruskin*; Forbes (2000), *The Legacy of John Ruskin and an Introduction to Unto This Last*.

12. De Sylva (1981), *John Ruskin's Modern Painters I and II*.

13. Myerson (2000), *Transcendentalism*.

14. MacDougall (1990), *James Fenimore Cooper*; Mnassar (2015), *Competing Environmental Ethics in Cooper's 'The Pioneers'*; Wuntu (2014), *James Fenimore Cooper and the Idea of Environmental Conservation in the Leatherstocking Tales*.

15. Cooper (1823), *The Pioneers, or the Sources of the Susquehanna*, 292 paraphrased.

16. Gura (2007), *American Transcendentalism*, Myerson (2000), *Transcendentalism*

17. Emerson (1918), *The Early Years of the Saturday Club*.

18. For additional information see: Anonymous (1858), *American Country Life*; Anonymous (1859), *Hints to American Artists*; Durand (1855), *Letters on Landscape Painting. No. 1*.

19. Novak (1980), *Nature and Culture*.

20. Durand (1855), *Letters on Landscape Painting. No. 1*.

21. Howat (2005), *Frederic Church*; Novak (1980), *Nature and Culture*.

22. Stillman (1901), *The Autobiography of a Journalist*.

23. Stillman (1901), *The Autobiography of a Journalist*, 191.

24. Schlett (2015), *A Not Too Greatly Changed Eden*.

25. Dilsaver (2016), *America's National Park System*; Myerson (2000), *Transcendentalism*; Wuntu (2014), *James Fenimore Cooper and the Idea of Environmental Conservation in the Leatherstocking Tales*.

26. Ferber (2008), *An American Pre-Raphaelite in New York.*

27. DeLue (2004), *George Inness and the Science of Landscape.*

Chapter 2. Vacating the City

1. Myers (1988), *The Catskills.*

2. Egerton (2007), *A History of the Ecological Sciences, Part 25.*

3. Myers (1988), The *Catskills*; Stradling (2007), *Making Mountains.*

4. Stradling (2007), *Making Mountains*; Weiss (2004), *Tourism in America Before World War II.*

5. Oplinger and Halma (2006), *The Poconos*; Squeri (2002), *Better in the Poconos.*

6. Holson (2019), *The Catskills are Back.*

7. Perrottet (2013), *Where was the Birthplace of the American Vacation?*

8. Murray (1869), *Adventures in the Wilderness.*

9. Murray (1869), *Adventures in the Wilderness*, 9–12.

10. Gilborn (1981), *Durant*; Kaiser (1982), *Great Camps of the Adirondacks.*

11. Donaldson (1921), *A History of the Adirondacks.*

12. Perrottet (2013), *Where was the Birthplace of the American Vacation?*

13. Weiss (2004), *Tourism in America Before World War II.*

14. Weiss (2004), *Tourism in America Before World War II.*

15. Spaulding (1858), *Guide and Historical Relics of the White Mountains*; Willey and Thompson (1870), *History of the White Mountains.*

16. Dickerman (2013), *White Mountains Hiking History.*

17. Chamberlin (2016), *On the Trail.*

18. Ruskin (1990), *Thomas Cole and the White Mountains.*

19. Kilbourne (1916), *Chronicles of the White Mountains*; Weiss (2004), *Tourism in America Before World War II.*

20. Brown (1995), *Inventing New England*; Weiss (2004), *Tourism in America Before World War II.*

21. Tolles (1998), *The Grand Resort Hotels of the White Mountains.*

22. Spaulding (1858), *Guide and Historical Relics of the White Mountains*, 71–72.

23. Weiss (2004), *Tourism in America Before World War II.*

24. Nye (2020), *Hiking in America.*

25. Chamberlin (2016), *On the Trail*; Harper (2019), *The Ladies Merely Breathed Deeply*; Nye (2020), *Hiking in America.*

26. Emblidge (1996), *The Appalachian Trail Reader.*

27. MacKaye (1921), *An Appalachian Trail*, 7.

28. Marra (2021), *The Work Ahead.*

29. Bryson (1998), *A Walk in the Woods.*

30. Goldenberg *et al.* (2008), *Why Individuals Hike the Appalachian Trail.*

31. NPF (2021), *The Hike of a Lifetime.*

32. ATC (2021), *Media Room.*

33. Goldenberg *et al.* (2008), *Why Individuals Hike the Appalachian Trail.*

34. Goldenberg *et al.* (2008), *Why Individuals Hike the Appalachian Trail.*

35. Sullivan (2021), *Why I Hike.*

36. Seagren (2021), *Why I Hike.*

37. CDTC (2021), *History of the Continental Divide Trail.*

38. CDTC (2021), *History of the Continental Divide Trail.*

Chapter 3. Restorative Places for the Masses

1. Andreski (1968), *Military Organization and Society*; Marwick (1968), *The Impact of the First World War on British Society*.

2. Cook (2003), *Civil War America*.

3. Twain and Warner (1873), *The Gilded Age*.

4. McKnight-Nichols and Unger (2017), *Introduction Gilded Excesses*; Richardson (2017), *Reconstructing the Gilded Age and Progressive Era*.

5. Atack and Bateman (1992), *How Long was the Workday in 1880?*; Weeks (1883), *Report on the Statistics of Wages in Manufacturing Industries 1880*.

6. Cook (2003), *Civil War America*.

7. Riis (1890), *How the Other Half Lives*; Tarbell (1902), *Miss Tarbell's History of the Standard Oil Company*; Wetmore and Steffens (1902), *Tweed Days in St. Louis*.

8. Kennedy (1975), *Overview The Progressive Era*; Voss and Sherman (2000), *Breaking the Iron Law of Oligarchy*.

9. Forbath (1989), *The Shaping of the American Labor Movement*; Jones (1986), *Workers at Play*; Lenger (1991), *Beyond Exceptionalism*; Voss and Sherman (2000), *Breaking the Iron Law of Oligarchy*.

10. Adler (2006), *The Past as Prologue?*; Cornfield (1991), *The US Labor Movement*; Whaples (2001), *Hours of Work in U.S. History*.

11. Forbath (1989), *The Shaping of the American Labor Movement*.

12. Whaples (2001), *Hours of Work in U.S. History*.

13. Adler (2006), *The Past as Prologue?*; Forbath (1989), *The Shaping of the American Labor Movement*; Whaples (2001), *Hours of Work in U.S. History*.

14. Cornfield (1991), *The US Labor Movement*.

15. Fogel (2000), *The Fourth Great Awakening & the Future of Egalitarianism*.

16. Adler (2006), *The Past as Prologue?*; Forbath (1989), *The Shaping of the American Labor Movement*.

17. Fogel (2000), *The Fourth Great Awakening & the Future of Egalitarianism*; Whaples (2001), *Hours of Work in U.S. History*.

18. Colby and Ortman (2014), *The Baby Boom Cohort in the United States*; Frey and DeVol (2000), *America's Demography in the New Century*.

19. Jensen and Guthrie (2006), *Outdoor Recreation in America*; Shivers and deLisle (1997), *The Story of Leisure*.

20. Fogel (2000), *The Fourth Great Awakening & the Future of Egalitarianism*.

21. Fogel (2000), *The Fourth Great Awakening & the Future of Egalitarianism*.

22. Brooke (2008), *Ford Model T*.

23. Weiss (2004), *Tourism in America Before World War II*.

24. Melder (1960), *The "Tin Lizzie's" Golden Anniversary*.

25. Ford (1922), *My Life and Work*, 73.

26. Brooke (2008), *Ford Model T*; Melder (1960), *The "Tin Lizzie's" Golden Anniversary*; Onion *et al.* (2010), *Model T.*; Stephenson (1989), *Secrets of the Model T*. The mass-produced, private automobile earned the nickname *"Tin Lizzie"* because of its lightweight

design and sturdy steel construction. "Lizzie" was a common slang term for a horse or mule. The moniker gained widespread use after Noel Bullock raced his Model T Ford in the 1922 Pikes Peak road race. After completing the race, his "*Old Liz*" was so beat up that people compared it to a tin can. Yet, the name stuck especially since Bullock's car won the race beating more expensive cars available at the time.

27. Carter-Lome (2021), *The Rise and Fall of the American Roadside Motel*; Jakle (1981), *Touring by Automobile in 1932*; Melder (1960), *The "Tin Lizzie's" Golden Anniversary.*

28. Young (2017), *Heading Out.*

29. Weiss (2004), *Tourism in America Before World War II.*

30. USDOT (2022), *History of the Federal Highway Administration.*

31. Payne and Hurt (2024), *The Making of an American Cultural Icon.*

32. Wallis (2001), *Route 66.*

33. Jakle and Sculle (2008), *Motoring.*

34. Carter-Lome (2021), *The Rise and Fall of the American Roadside Motel*; Weingroff (1996), *Federal-Aid Highway Act of 1956.*

35. USDOT (2022), *History of the Federal Highway Administration.*

36. Bell (2008), *Design for Outdoor Recreation.*

37. Nye (2020), *Hiking in America.*

38. Carter-Lome (2021), *The Rise and Fall of the American Roadside Motel.*

39. Gibbens (2017), *Creepy Photos Show Abandoned American Resort Towns*; Holson (2019), *The Catskills are Back*; Strochlic (2022), *Borscht Belt Revisited.*

40. Jakle (1981), *Touring by Automobile in 1932.*

41. Zierer (1952), *Tourism and Recreation in the West*, 481.

42. Weiss (2004), *Tourism in America Before World War II.*

43. Leonard and Noel (1990), *Denver.*

44. Leonard and Noel (1990), *Denver.*

45. Fielder *et al.* (2013), *Denver Mountain Parks*, 14.

46. Rex-Atzet (2011), *Denver's Mountain Playground*; Fiore (2018), *Morrison History.*

47. Fielder *et al.* (2013), *Denver Mountain Parks*,138.

48. Downing (1931), *How Denver Acquired Her Celebrated Mountain Parks.*

49. Downing (1931), *How Denver Acquired Her Celebrated Mountain Parks*, 14.

50. Baird and Bishop (2008), *Denver Mountain Parks Master Plan 2008*; Downing (1931), *How Denver Acquired Her Celebrated Mountain Parks.*

51. Rex-Atzet (2011), *Denver's Mountain Playground.*

52. Rex-Atzet (2011), *Denver's Mountain Playground.*

53. Downing (1931), *How Denver Acquired Her Celebrated Mountain Parks.*

54. Downing (1931), *How Denver Acquired Her Celebrated Mountain Parks.*

55. Downing (1931), *How Denver Acquired Her Celebrated Mountain Parks*, 23.

56. Fielder *et al.* (2013), *Denver Mountain Parks.*

57. LandScope (2021), *Open Space 101.*

58. Brown and Wardwell (1980), *New Directions in Urban-Rural Migration*; Ford (1999), *Understanding Population Growth in the Peri-Urban Region.*

59. Schmidt (2008), *The Evolving Relationship Between Open Space Preservation and Local Planning Practice*; Stanley *et al.* (2012), *Urban Open Spaces in Historical Perspective.*

60. JCOS (2020*a*), *Jefferson County Open Space*.

61. Hoby (2014), *Jefferson County Open Space*.

62. JCOS (2020*a*), *Jefferson County Open Space*.

63. JCOS (2020*b*), *Jeffco Trails Plan*.

64. Kennedy (2018), *Resident Survey 2018*.

65. Hoby (2014), *Jefferson County Open Space*.

66. Kennedy (2018), *Resident Survey 2018*.

67. JCOS (2020*b*), *Jeffco Trails Plan*.

68. Baird and Bishop (2008), *Denver Mountain Parks Master Plan 2008*.

69. Meyer (2021), *Good News, Hikers*.

70. Rex-Atzet (2020), *Denver Mountain Parks*.

71. Baird and Bishop (2008), *Denver Mountain Parks Master Plan 2008*.

72. Downing (1931), *How Denver Acquired Her Celebrated Mountain Parks*; Baird and Bishop (2008), *Denver Mountain Parks Master Plan 2008*.

73. HC (2021), *Denver Mountain Parks*.

74. Baird and Bishop (2008), *Denver Mountain Parks Master Plan 2008*, 155.

75. Fielder *et al.* (2013), *Denver Mountain Parks*, 64.

Chapter 4. Nature in the City

1. Gibson (2024), *American Demographic History Chartbook*.

2. Hall (1984), *The Organization of American Culture 1700–1900*.

3. Jefferson (1829), *Notes on the State of Virginia*; Peterson (1991), *Telling the Farmers' Story*.

4. Ruggles (2015), *Patriarchy, Power, and Pay*.

5. Hall (1984), *The Organization of American Culture 1700–1900*.

6. Baics and Meisterlin (2016), *Zoning Before Zoning*; Kennedy (1992), *Planning the City Upon a Hill*.

7. Riis (1890), *How the Other Half Lives*.

8. Song *et al.* (2016), *Physiological Effects of Nature Therapy*.

9. Beaujeu-Garnier (1984), *Urbanism and Large Cities*.

10. Stanley *et al.* (2012), *Urban Open Spaces in Historical Perspective*.

11. Rudd-Jones (2015), *A Brief History of Urban Green Spaces*.

12. McLean and Hurd (2015), *Kraus' Recreation and Leisure in Modern Society*.

13. Batey (1994), *The Picturesque*; Brook (2008), *Wildness in the English Garden Tradition*.

14. Rex-Atzet (2011), *Denver's Mountain Playground*.

15. McLean and Hurd (2015), *Kraus' Recreation and Leisure in Modern Society*.

16. McLean and Hurd (2015), *Kraus' Recreation and Leisure in Modern Society*, 43.

17. Fisher (2011), *Nature in the City*.

18. Beveridge (2023), *Frederick Law Olmsted*; Rybczynski (1999), *A Clearing in the Distance*.

19. Fisher (2011), *Nature in the City*; Kang (2017), *160 Years of Central Park*.

20. Fisher (2011), *Nature in the City*; Rosenzweig and Blackmar (1992), *The Park and the People*.

21. U.S. Census (2022), *Manhattan Borough.*

22. C.P. (2018), *Central Park FAQ*; Statista (2022), *City Parks in the U.S. by Annual Visitorship in 2020*; van Buren (2016), *12 Secrets of New York's Central Park.*

23. Kang (2017), *160 Years of Central Park.*

24. Kang (2017), *160 Years of Central Park*; Nowak (2002), *The Effects of Urban Trees on Air Quality.*

25. Lawless, Loughlin, and Meier (2008), *The Master List of Design Projects of the Olmsted Firm.*

26. Beveridge (2021), *The Seven S's of Olmsted Design.*

27. Rybczynski (1999), *A Clearing in the Distance.*

28. Olmsted and Roper (1952), *The Yosemite Valley and the Mariposa Big Trees*, 21.

29. Beveridge (2023), *Frederick Law Olmsted.*

30. Beveridge *et al.* (2015), *Frederick Law Olmsted*, xiii.

31. Young (2018), *Frederick Law Olmsted's Abandoned San Francisco Park Plan*; Zeller (2022), *Consuming Landscapes.*

32. Riis (1890), *How the Other Half Lives.*

33. Fairfield (2018), *The City Beautiful Movement.*

34. Fairfield (2018), *The City Beautiful Movement*, 3.

35. Fairfield (2018), *The City Beautiful Movement.*

36. Smith (2009), *Taming the Savage City*, 8–9.

37. Rex-Atzet (2011), *Denver's Mountain Playground.*

38. VisitKC (2022), *Super Cities.*

39. Fairfield (2018), *The City Beautiful Movement.*

40. McLean and Hurd (2015), *Kraus' Recreation and Leisure in Modern Society.*

41. Rex-Atzet (2011), *Denver's Mountain Playground.*

42. McLean and Hurd (2015), *Kraus' Recreation and Leisure in Modern Society.*

Chapter 5. Sanctuaries of Healing

1. Nash (1989), *The Rights of Nature*; Worster (1994), *The Wealth of Nature.*

2. Muir (1898), *The Wild Parks and Forest Reservations of the West*, various.

3. Rowthorn (2012), *The Wisdom of John Muir*; Teale (1954), *The Wilderness World of John Muir.*

4. Muir (1901), *Our National Parks*, 56.

5. Fagan (2001), *The Genesis of the Roman Public Bath.*

6. Bowman (1998), *Belief, Legend and Perceptions of the Sacred in Contemporary Bath.*

7. UNESCO (2021), *The Great Spa Towns of Europe.*

8. Gianfaldoni *et al.* (2017), *History of the Baths and Thermal Medicine.*

9. NPS (2020), *Hot Springs National Park Arkansas.*

10. Paige and Harrison (1988), *Out of the Vapors.*

11. Hill (2014), *Hot Springs National Park.*

12. Carpenter (2019), *"Cesspools," Springs, and Snaking Pipes.*

13. Carpenter (2019), *"Cesspools," Springs, and Snaking Pipes*; NPS (2020), *Hot Springs National Park Arkansas.*

14. Barger (2021), *Feeling Frazzled?*

15. NPS (2020), *Hot Springs National Park Arkansas*.

16. NPS (2020), *Hot Springs National Park Arkansas*.

17. NPS (2020), *Hot Springs National Park Arkansas*; Schmalz *et al.* (2013), *Development of a Healthy Parks Healthy People Strategic Action Plan for Hot Springs National Park*.

18. Hill (2014), *Hot Springs National Park*.

19. NPS (2020), *Hot Springs National Park Arkansas*.

20. Hill (2014), *Hot Springs National Park*.

21. NPS (2020), *Hot Springs National Park Arkansas*.

22. Barberis *et al.* (2017), *The History of Tuberculosis*; Daniel (2006), *The History of Tuberculosis*.

23. Barberis *et al.* Barberis *et al.* (2017), *The History of Tuberculosis*; Blakemore (2020),*The Disease that Helped Put Colorado on the Map*.

24. Keers (1980), *Two Forgotten Pioneers*.

25. Kanabus (2020), *Sanatorium*.

26. Daniel (2006), *The History of Tuberculosis*; Kanabus (2020), *Sanatorium*.

27. Grineski *et al.* (2006), *Tuberculosis and Urban Growth*; Neufeld (2019), *Visiting Our Past*.

28. Daniel (2006), *The History of Tuberculosis*.

29. CDC (2016), *Tuberculosis (TB)*.

30. Luce (2014), *The White Plague in the City of Angels*; Rothman (1994), *Living in the Shadow of Death*.

31. CDC (2016), *Tuberculosis (TB)*; Glaser and Johnston (1954), *Index of Hospitals and Sanatoria with Tuberculosis Beds in the United States*.

32. Harner (2021), *Profiting from the Peak*, 52.

33. Abel (2007), *Tuberculosis and the Politics of Exclusion*; Hart (2012), *When Lungers Came to Tucson*; Jones (1966), *A Burden on the Southwest*; Rothman (1994), *Living in the Shadow of Death*.

34. Jones (1966), *A Burden on the Southwest*.

35. Grineski *et al.* (2006), *Tuberculosis and Urban Growth*.

36. Hodge (1877), *Arizona As It Is*, 28–29.

37. Abel (2007), *Tuberculosis and the Politics of Exclusion*; Jones (1966), *A Burden on the Southwest*; Rothman (1994), *Living in the Shadow of Death*.

38. Hart (2012), *When Lungers Came to Tucson*.

39. Jones (1966), *A Burden on the Southwest*.

40. Grineski *et al.* (2006), *Tuberculosis and Urban Growth*; Hart (2012), *When Lungers Came to Tucson*.

41. Glaser and Johnston (1954), *Index of Hospitals and Sanatoria with Tuberculosis Beds in the United States*.

42. Glaser and Johnston (1954), *Index of Hospitals and Sanatoria with Tuberculosis Beds in the United States*; Jones (1966), *A Burden on the Southwest*.

43. Iddings (1896), *Life in the Altitudes*.

44. Blakemore (2020), *The Disease that Helped Put Colorado on the Map*; Stout (1997), *A Consumptives' Refuge*.

45. Jones (1966), *A Burden on the Southwest*.

46. Blakemore (2020), *The Disease that Helped Put Colorado on the Map;* Harner (2021), *Profiting from the Peak.*

47. Harner (2021), *Profiting from the Peak*, 53.

48. McKay (1979), *A History of the Nordrach Ranch.*

49. Fallon (1992), *Health & History*; Stout (1997), *A Consumptives' Refuge.*

50. McKay (1979), *A History of the Nordrach Ranch*, 179.

51. Stout (1997), *A Consumptives' Refuge.*

52. Jones (1966), *A Burden on the Southwest.*

53. Daniel (2006), *The History of Tuberculosis*; Kanabus (2020), *Sanatorium.*

54. Callaghan *et al.* (2021), *Feeling Good*; Chandrashekhar (2022), *Can the 19th-century Health Practice Help with Long COVID?*; Goodall (2022), *The Rise of Wellness Tourism*; Hekmat *et al.* (2021), *Wellness Tourism Experience on the Rise Post COVID.*

Conclusion: Lessons from the Past

1. Alvarez *et al.* (2022), *A Review of Nature Deficit Disorder*; Sparling *et al.* (2000) *Promoting Physical Activity*; Turner et *al.* (2004) *Global Urbanization and the Separation of Humans from Nature.*

2. Quinn and Helmstetter (2019), *How Often do Americans Spend Free Time in Nature.*

3. Williams (2016), *This is Your Brain on Nature.*

4. Leonhardt (2022), *On the Phone, Alone*; Seo (2023), *America is Getting Lonelier and More Indoorsy.*

5. Bratman *et al.* (2015), *Nature Experience Reduces Rumination and Subgenual Prefrontal Cortex Activation*; Palomino et *al.* (2016), *The Online Dissemination of Nature-Health Concepts*; Townsend *et al.* (2018), *Therapeutic Landscapes, Restorative Environments, Place Attachment, and Well-being*; Wang et *al.* (2023), *The Role of Nature-Deficit Disorder in the Associations Between Mobile Phone Overuse and Well-being and Mindfulness*; WHO (2019), *Mental Disorders Fact Sheet.*

6. Louv (2005), *Last Child in the Woods.*

7. Pratt and Brody (2008), *Depression in the United States Household Population;* Witters (2023), *U.S. Depression Rates Reach New High.*

8. Grathwohl (2024), *Oxford Word of the Year 2024*; Ortiz-Ospina (2019), *The Rise of Social Media.*

9. Harris *et al.* (2025), *The State of the Nation.*

10. Bittel (2023), *Noise Pollution Harms More Than Your Hearing*; Goines and Hagler (2007), *Noise Pollution*; Ikonte et *al.* (2020), *Trends in Prevalence of Depression and Serious Psychological Distress in the United States*; Kinnealey and Fuiek (1999), *The Relationship Between Sensory Defensiveness Anxiety, Depression and Perception of Pain in Adults*; Kramer (2010), *The Effects of Psychological Torture*; Liss et *al.* (2008), *The Relationships Between Sensory Processing Sensitivity, Alexithymia, Autism, Depression, and Anxiety*; MacKerron and Mourato (2013), *Happiness is Greater in Natural Environments*; Scheydt et *al.* (2017), *Review Article Sensory Overload.*

11. Ilardi (2009), *The Depression Cure*; Lederbogen *et al.* (2011), *City Living and Urban Upbringing Affect Neural Social Stress Processing in Humans.*

12. Berto (2005), *Exposure to Restorative Environments Help Restore Attentional Capacity*; Hartig et *al.* (1997), *A Measure of Restorative Quality in Environments*; Herzog

et al. (2003), *Assessing the Restorative Components of Environments*; Kaplan (1995), *The Restorative Benefits of Nature*.

13. Bell *et al.* (2018), *From Therapeutic Landscapes to Healthy Spaces, Places and Practices*; Gesler (1992), *Therapeutic Landscapes*; Williams (1999), *Therapeutic Landscapes*.

14. Bell *et al.* (2023), *From Therapeutic Landscape to Therapeutic 'Sensescape' Experiences with Nature*.

15. Kaplan and Kaplan (1989), *The Experience of Nature*.

16. Berto (2014), *The Role of Nature in Coping with Psycho-Physiological Stress*; Hartig (2011), *Issues in Restorative Environments Research*; Hartig *et al.* (1997), *A Measure of Restorative Quality in Environments*; Hartig *et al.* (2014), *Nature and Health*; Herzog et al. (2003), *Assessing the Restorative Components of Environments*; Scopelliti *et al.* (2019), *Is it Really Nature that Restores People?*

17. Bell *et al.* (2018), *From Therapeutic Landscapes to Healthy Spaces, Places and Practices*; Cattell *et al.* (2008), *Mingling, Observing, and Lingering*; Gesler (1996), *Lourdes*; Williams (2007), *Therapeutic Landscapes*.

18. Bell *et al.* (2023), *From Therapeutic Landscape to Therapeutic 'Sensescape' Experiences with Nature*; Doughty (2019), *Therapeutic Landscapes*; Mossabir *et al.* (2021), *Therapeutic Landscape Experiences of Everyday Geographies within the Wider Community*.

19. Hartig (2011), *Issues in Restorative Environments Research*; Kellert *et al.* (2008), *Biophilic Design*; Townsend *et al.* (2018), *Therapeutic Landscapes, Restorative Environments, Place Attachment, and Well-being*.

20. Barbieri and Rossero (2024), *It Is Like Post-Traumatic Stress Disorder*.

21. Ulrich (1984), *View Through a Window May Influence Recovery from Surgery*.

22. Berto (2014), *The Role of Nature in Coping with Psycho-Physiological Stress*; Carr (2021), *Topography of Wellness*; Kandola et al. (2019), *Physical Activity and Depression*; Kuo and Taylor (2004), *A Potential Natural Treatment for Attention-Deficit Hyperactivity Disorder*; Maller *et al.* (2005), *Healthy Nature Healthy People*; Song *et al.* (2016), *Physiological Effects of Nature Therapy*; Walker (2004), *The Public Value of Urban Parks*.

23. Hartig (2011), *Issues in Restorative Environments Research*, 44.

24. Bullock *et al.* (2018), *An Exploration of the Relationships Between Cultural Ecosystem Services, Socio-cultural Values and Well being*; Huynh *et al.* (2022), *Linking the Nonmaterial Dimensions of Human-Nature Relations*; Kosanic and Petzold (2020), *A Systematic Review of Cultural Ecosystem Services and Human Wellbeing*; McMichael *et al.* (2005), *Linking Ecosystem Services and Human Well-being*.

25. Muir (1901), *Our National Parks*, 1.

26. Chamberlin (2016), *On the Trail*; Emblidge (1996), *The Appalachian Trail Reader*; Nye (2020), *Hiking in America*.

27. Hartig (2011), *Issues in Restorative Environments Research*; Herzog et al. (2003), *Assessing the Restorative Components of Environments*; Kaplan and Kaplan (1989), *The Experience of Nature*.

28. Harner (2021), *Profiting from the Peak*.

29. Callaghan *et al.* (2021), *Feeling Good*; Chandrashekhar (2022), *Can the 19th-Century Health Practice Help with Long COVID?*; Goodall (2022), *The Rise of Wellness Tourism*; Hekmat *et al.* (2021), *Wellness Tourism Experience on the Rise Post COVID*.

30. Aman (2022), *Amangiri*.

31. Jensen and Guthrie (2006), *Outdoor Recreation in America*.

32. Browning and Ryan (2020), *Nature Inside*; Kellert *et al.* (2008), *Biophilic Design*; Roe and McCay (2021), *Restorative Cities*.

33. Armato (2017), *Pocket Parks*; Larson *et al.* (2013), *Beyond Restoration and into Design*; Peschardt and Stigsdotter (2013), *Associations Between Park Characteristics and Perceived Restorativeness of Small Public Urban Garden Spaces*.

34. Jensen and Guthrie (2006), *Outdoor Recreation in America*.

35. FPC (2024), *Experience Forest Park*.

36. Quinn and Helmstetter (2019), *How Often do Americans Spend Free Time in Nature*.

37. White *et al.* (2016), *Federal Outdoor Recreation Trends*; Winter *et al.* (2020), *Outdoor Recreation, Nature-Based Tourism, and Sustainability*.

38. Carr and Williams (1993), *Understanding the Role of Ethnicity in Outdoor Recreation Experiences*; Ryan *et al.* (2020), *Engaging Minority Communities in Local National Park Units*; Weber and Sultana (2013), *Why Do So Few Minority People Visit National Parks?*

39. Quinn and Helmstetter (2019), *How Often do Americans Spend Free Time in Nature*.

40. Reese and Myers (2012), *EcoWellness*; Reese *et al.* (2019), *EcoWellness*.

41. Baird and Bishop (2008) *Denver Mountain Parks Master Plan 2008*; Kennedy (2018), *Resident Survey 2018*.

42. Bellamy (2021), *Wilderness on Wheels*; Zimmerman, (2021), *This Park County Camp is a Prime Example of Accessibility in Nature*.

43. Cresswell (2004), *Place*; Lewicka (2011), *Place Attachment*; Low and Altman (1992), *Place Attachment*; Manzo and Devine-Wright (2014), *Place Attachment*; Scannell and Gifford (2014), *Defining Place Attachment*; Seamon (2014), *Place Attachment and Phenomenology*; Tuan (1977), *Space and Place*.

44. Smith (2018), *Explorations in Place Attachment*.

References and Further Readings

Abel, E. K. 2007. *Tuberculosis and the Politics of Exclusion: A History of Public Health and Migration to Los Angeles*. New Brunswick: Rutgers University Press.

Adler, J. 2006. The Past as Prologue?: A Brief History of the Labor Movement in the United States. *Public Personnel Management* 35 (4): 311–329.

Alban, D. 2016. Overstimulation: Taming a Modern Problem that Leads to Anxiety. *Reset Me*. http://reset.me/story/overstimulation-taming-a-modern-problem-that-leads-to-anxiety/.

Alvarez, E., A. Garcia, and P. Le. 2022. A Review of Nature Deficit Disorder (NDD) and its Disproportionate Impacts on Latinx Populations. *Environmental Development* 43: 100732–100739.

Aman. 2022. Amangiri. [https://www.aman.com/resorts/amangiri].

Anderson, J., K. Ruggeri, K. Steemers, and F. Huppert. 2017. Lively Social Space, Well-Being Activity, and Urban Design: Findings from a Low-Cost Community-Led Public Space Intervention. *Environment & Behavior* 49 (6): 685–716.

Andreski, S. 1968. *Military Organization and Society*. Berkeley: University of California Press.

Andrews, G. 2004. (Re)thinking the Dynamics Between Healthcare and Place: Therapeutic Geographies in Treatment and Care Practices. *Area* 36 (3): 307–318.

Anonymous. 1858. American Country Life. *The Crayon* 5 (10): 279–281.

Anonymous. 1859. Hints to American Artists. *The Crayon* 6 (5): 145–146.

Appalachian Trail Conservancy (ATC). 2021. *Media Room*. [https://appalachiantrail.org/our-work/about-us/media-room/].

Armato, F. 2017. Pocket Park: Product Urban Design. *The Design Journal* 20 (1): 1869–1878.

Atack, J. and F. Bateman. 1992. How Long Was the Workday in 1880? *Journal of Economic History* 52 (1): 129–160.

Ayres, A. J. 1979. *Sensory Integration and the Child*. Los Angeles: Western Psychological Services.

Bagot, K., F. Kuo, and F. Allen. 2007. Amendments to the Perceived Restorative Components Scale for Children (PRCS-C II). *Children Youth and Environments* 17: 124–127.

Baics, G. and L. Meisterlin. 2016. Zoning Before Zoning: Land Use and Density in Mid-Nineteenth-Century New York City. *Annals of the American Association of Geographers* 106 (5): 1152–1175.

Baird, S. and T. Bishop. 2008. *Denver Mountain Parks Master Plan 2008*. Denver: Denver Parks and Recreation. [https://www.denvergov.org/files/assets/public/parks-and-recreation/documents/planning/mountainpark_masterplan.pdf].

Barberis, I., N. L. Bragazzi, L. Galluzzo, and M. Martini. 2017. The History of Tuberculosis: From the First Historical Records to the Isolation of Koch's Bacillus. *Journal of Preventive Medicine and Hygiene* 58 (1): 9–12.

Barbieri, A. and E. Rossero. 2024. "It is Like Post-Traumatic Stress Disorder, but in a Positive Sense!: New Territories of the Self as Inner Therapeutic Landscapes for Youth Experiencing Mental Ill-Health." *Health and Place* 85: 103157. [https://doi.org/10.1016/j.healthplace.2023.103157].

Barger, J. 2021. Feeling Frazzled? These Soothing Hot Springs Let You Unwind: Find Healing Waters Around the U.S., From Natural Pools in the West to a Historic Arkansas Spa Town. *National Geographic*, 11 March. [https://www.nationalgeographic.com/travel/article/feeling-frazzled-these-soothing-hot- springs-let-you-unwind].

Barnett, R. 2012. John Muir and "Godful" Nature. *Religions* 3 266–288.

Batey, M. 1994. The Picturesque: An Overview. *Garden History* 22 (2): 121–132.

Beatley T. 2016. *Handbook of Biophilic City Planning and Design*. Washington, DC: Island Press.

Beaujeu-Garnier, J. 1984. Urbanism and Large Cities: The Parisian Experience. *Urban Geography* 5 (4): 292–307.

Bell, S. 2008. *Design for Outdoor Recreation*. New York: Taylor & Francis.

Bell, S., B. Wheeler, and C. Phoenix. 2017. Using Geonarratives to Explore the Diverse Temporalities of Therapeutic Landscapes: Perspectives from "Green" and "Blue" Settings. *Annals of the American Association of Geographers* 107 (1): 93–108.

Bell, S., C. Hickman, and F. Houghton. 2023. From Therapeutic Landscape to Therapeutic 'Sensescape' Experiences with Nature? A Scoping Review. *Wellbeing, Space and Society* 4: 100126. [doi.org/10.1016/j.wss.2022.100126].

Bell, S., R. Foley, F. Houghton, A. Maddrell, and A. Williams. 2018. From Therapeutic Landscapes to Healthy Spaces, Places and Practices: A Scoping Review. *Social Science and Medicine* 196 (1): 123–130.

Bellamy, B. 2021. *Wilderness on Wheels*. [https://www.wildernessonwheels.org/].

Berto, R. 2005. Exposure to Restorative Environments Helps Restore Attentional Capacity. *Journal of Environmental Psychology* 25: 249–259.

Berto, R. 2014. The Role of Nature in Coping with Psycho-Physiological Stress: A Literature Review of Restorativeness. *Behavioral Sciences* 4: 394–409.

Berto, R. and G. Barbiero. 2017. The Biophilic Quality Index: A Tool to Improve a Building "Green" to Restorative. *Visions for Sustainability* 8: 38–45.

Berto, R., G. Barbiero, M. Pasini, and P. Unema. 2014. Biophilic Design Triggers Fascination and Enhances Psychological Restoration in the Urban Environment. *Journal of Biourbanism* 1/2: 27–34.

Beveridge, C. 2021. *The Seven S's of Olmsted Design*. [https://olmsted.org/the-seven-ss-of-olmsted-design/].

Beveridge, C. 2023. *Frederick Law Olmsted: His Essential Theory*. [https://olmsted.org/frederick-law-olmsted-his-essential-theory/].

Beveridge, C., L. Meier, and I. Mills 2015. *Frederick Law Olmsted: Plans and Views of Public Parks*. Baltimore: Johns Hopkins University Press.

Bittel, J. 2023. Noise Pollution Harms More Than Your Hearing. *National Geographic*, 7 November.

Blake, K. 2001. Contested Landscapes of Navajo Sacred Mountains. *North American Geographer* 3 (1): 29–62.

Blakemore, E. 2020. *The Disease That Helped Put Colorado on the Map*. A&E Television Networks, LLC [https://www.history.com/news/the-disease-that-helped-put-colorado-on-the-map].

Blewitt, J. 2019. *William Morris & John Ruskin: A New Road on Which the World Should Travel*. Exeter: University of Exeter Press.

Bodin, M. and T. Hartig. 2003. Does the Outdoor Environment Matter for Psychological Restoration Gained Through Running? *Psychology of Sport and Exercise* 4: 141–153.

Bowman, M. 1998. Belief, Legend and Perceptions of the Sacred in Contemporary Bath. *Folklore* 109: 25–31.

Bratman, G. N., J. P. Hamilton, K. S. Hahn, G. C. Daily, and J. J. Gross. 2015. Nature Experience Reduces Rumination and Subgenual Prefrontal Cortex Activation. *Proceedings of the National Academy of Sciences* 112 (28): 8567–8572.

Brewster, L. 2014. The Public Library as Therapeutic Landscape: A Qualitative Case Study. *Health & Place* 26 (1): 94–99.

Brook, I. 2008. Wildness in the English Garden Tradition: A Reassessment of the Picturesque from Environmental Philosophy. *Ethics and the Environment* 13 (1): 105–119.

Brooke, L. 2008. *Ford Model T: The Car That Put the World on Wheels*. Minneapolis, MN: MBI Publishing Co.

Brown, D. 1995. *Inventing New England: Regional Tourism in the Nineteenth Century*. Washington, D.C.: Smithsonian Institution Press.

Brown, D. L. and J. M. Wardwell. 1980. *New Directions in Urban-Rural Migration: The Population Turnaround in Rural America*. New York: Academic Press.

Browning W. and C. Ryan. 2020. *Nature Inside: A Biophilic Design Guide*. New York: Routledge.

Brunn, S., D. J. Zeigler, M. Hays-Mitchell, and J. K. Graybill. 2020. *Cities of the World: Regional Patterns and Urban Environments*. London: Rowman & Littlefield.

Bryson, B. 1998. *A Walk in the Woods: Rediscovering America on the Appalachian Trail*. New York: Anchor Books.

Buell, L. 1995. *The Environmental Imagination: Thoreau, Nature Writing, and the Formation of American Culture*. Cambridge: Harvard University Press.

Buell, L. 2003. *Emerson*. Cambridge: Harvard University Press.

Bullock, C., D. Joyce, and M. Collier. 2018. An Exploration of the Relationships Between Cultural Ecosystem Services, Socio-cultural Values and Well-being. *Ecosystem Services* 31 (1): 142–152.

Buttimer, A. 1976. Grasping the Dynamism of Lifeworld. *Annals of the Association of American Geographers* 66 (2): 277–292.

Buttimer, A. and D. Seamon. 1980. *The Human Experience of Space and Place*. New York: Routledge.

Callaghan, S., M. Losch, A. Pione, and W. Teichner. 2021. Feeling Good: The Future of the $1.5 Trillion Wellness Market. *McKinsey & Company* 8 April. [https://www.mckinsey.com/industries/consumer-packaged-goods/our-insights/feeling-good-the-future-of-the-1-5-trillion-wellness-market?cid=other-eml-alt-mip- mck&hdpid=931d5f23-1699-42e3-a9e1- eba50cebdba3&hctky=2505496&hlkid=19600173076a471e930ef1abb#].

Carpenter, K. 2019. "Cesspools," Springs, and Snaking Pipes. *Technology's Stories* 7 (1): 1–14. [https://www.technologystories.org/cesspools-springs].

Carr, D. and D. Williams. 1993. Understanding the Role of Ethnicity in Outdoor Recreation Experiences. *Journal of Leisure Research* 25 (1): 22–38.

Carr, S. 2021. *The Topography of Wellness: How Health and Disease Shaped the American Landscape*. Charlottesville: University of Virginia Press.

Carrus, G., et al. 2017. A Different Way to Stay in Touch With 'Urban Nature': The Perceived Restorative Qualities of Botanical Gardens. *Frontiers in Psychology* 31 May. [https://www.frontiersin.org/articles/10.3389/fpsyg.2017.00914/full].

Carter-Lome, M. 2021. The Rise and Fall of the American Roadside Motel. *Journal of Antiques and Collectibles*, 10 May. [https://journalofantiques.com/digital-publications/joac-magazine/features/the/].

Cattell, V., N. Dines, W. Gesler, and S. Curtis. 2008. Mingling, Observing, and Lingering: Everyday Public Spaces and Their Implications for Well-being and Social Relations. *Health & Place* 14 (3): 544–561.

CDC [Centers for Disease Control]. 1999. Achievements in Public Health, 1900–1999: Control of Infectious Diseases. *Morbidity and Mortality Weekly Report* 48 (29): 621–629. [https://www.cdc.gov/mmwr/preview/mmwrhtml/mm4829a1.htm#:~:text=In%201900%2C%20the%20three%20leading,than%205%20years%20(1)].

CDC [Centers for Disease Control]. 2016. Tuberculosis (TB). *Centers for Disease Control and Prevention*, 12 December. [https://www.cdc.gov/tb/worldtbday/history.htm].

CDTC [Continental Divide Trail Conservancy]. 2021. *History of the Continental Divide Trail*. Golden, CO: Continental Divide Trail Coalition. [https://continentaldividetrail.org/history-of-the-cdt/].

Chamberlin, S. 2016. *On the Trail: A History of American Hiking*. New Haven: Yale University Press.

Chandrashekhar, V. 2022. Can the 19th-century Health Practice Help with Long COVID? *National Geographic* 8 April.

Clancy, J., and C. Ryan. 2015. The Role of Biophilic Design in Landscape Architecture for Health and Well-Being. *Landscape Architecture Frontiers* 3 (1): 54–61.

Colby, S. and J. Ortman. 2014. The Baby Boom Cohort in the United States: 2012 to 2060. *Current Population Reports, U.S. Bureau of the Census*. [https://www.census.gov/prod/2014pubs/p25-1141.pdf].

Cole, T. 1836. Essay on the American Scenery. *American Monthly Magazine* 7 (1): 1–12.

Collins, J. 2020. *The Architecture and Landscape of Health: A Historical Perspective on Therapeutic Places, 1790–1940*. London: Routledge.

Congdon, K. G., D. Blandy, and D. Coeyman. 2014. *Happy Clouds, Happy Trees: The Bob Ross Phenomenon*. Jackson: University Press of Mississippi.

Conradson, D. 2005. Landscape, Care and the Relational Self: Therapeutic Encounters in Rural England. *Health & Place* 11 (1): 337–348.

Cook, R. 2003. *Civil War America: Making a Nation, 1848–1877*. New York: Routledge.

Cooper, J. F. 1823. *The Pioneers, or the Sources of the Susquehanna; A Descriptive Tale*. New York: Charles Wiley.

Cornfield, D. 1991. The US Labor Movement: Its Development and Impact on Social Inequality and Politics. *Annual Review of Sociology* 17 (1): 27–49.

CP [Central Park]. 2018. *Central Park FAQ*. [https://centralpark.org/faq-2/].

Cresswell, T. 2004. *Place: A Short Introduction*. Oxford: Blackwell.

Cronon, W. 1996. The Trouble with Wilderness: Or, Getting Back to the Wrong Nature. *Environmental History* 1 (1): 7–28.

Curtis, K. 2010. The Virtue of Thoreau: Biography, Geography, and History in Walden Woods. *Environmental History* 15 (1): 31–53.

Cutler, P. 2009. Sutro Baths: Caracalla at Lands End. *Journal of the California Garden & Landscape History Society* 12 (1): 1–12.

Daniel, T. M. 2006. The History of Tuberculosis. *Respiratory Medicine* 100: 1862–1870.

Delgado, James P., Denise Bradley, Paul M. Scolari, and Stephen A. Haller. 2000. The History and Significance of the Adolph Sutro Historic District: Excerpts from the National Registry of Historic Places. *National Park Service*. [https://www.nps.gov/goga/learn/historyculture/upload/sutro_history.pdf].

Delistraty, C. 2019. The Happiness Ruse. *Aeon*. 31 October. [https://aeon.co/essays/how-did-being-happy-become-a-matter-of-relentless-competitive-work].

DeLue, R. Z. 2004. *George Inness and the Science of Landscape*. Chicago: University of Chicago Press.

De Sylva, G. 1981. *John Ruskin's Modern Painters I and II: A Phenomenological Analysis*. Ann Arbor: University of Michigan Research Press.

de Wit, C. 2003. Field Methods for Investigating Sense of Place. *North American Geographer* 5 (1): 5–30.

Dickerman, M. 2013. *White Mountains Hiking History: Trailblazers of the Granite State*. Charleston, SC: The History Press.

Dilsaver, L. 2016. *America's National Park System: The Critical Documents*. Lanham: Rowman & Littlefield.

Donaldson, A. 1921. *A History of the Adirondacks*. New York: The Century Company.

Doughty, K. 2019. Therapeutic Landscapes. In *The Routledge Companion to Landscape Studies*, edited by P. Howard, I. Thompson, E. Waterton, and M Atha, 341–353. London: Routledge.

Downing, W. 1931. How Denver Acquired Her Celebrated Mountain Parks. *Municipal Facts* March–April: 12–14, 23, 28.

Durand, A. B. 1855. Letters on Landscape Painting. No. 1. *The Crayon* 1 (1): 1–2.

Egerton, F. N. 2007. A History of the Ecological Sciences, Part 25, American Naturalists Explore Eastern North America: John and William Bartram. *Bulletin of the Ecological Society of America* 88 (3): 253–268.

Emblidge, D. 1996. *The Appalachian Trail Reader*. New York: Oxford University Press.

Emerson, R. W. 1836. *Nature*. Boston: James Munroe and Company.

Emerson, E. W. 1918. *The Early Years of the Saturday Club, 1855–1870*. Boston: Houghton Mifflin Co.

Fagan, G. G. 2001. The Genesis of the Roman Public Bath: Recent Approaches and Future Directions. *American Journal of Archaeology* 105 (3): 403–426.

Fairfield, J. D. 2018. *The City Beautiful Movement, 1890–1920*. Oxford: Oxford University Press.

Fallon, D. 1992. Health & History: Around Turn of Century, Tuberculosis Patients Sought Cure in Springs. *Colorado Springs Gazette Telegraph* 19 April: B1.

FDA [U.S. Food and Drug Administration]. 2019. Depression Medicines. *U.S. Food & Drug Administration*. 30 September. [https://www.fda.gov/consumers/free-publications-women/depression-medicines].

Ferber, L. S. 2008. An American Pre-Raphaelite in New York: William Trost Richards. *Archives of American Art Journal* 47(1): 4–15.

Fielder, J., W. Rex-Atzet, S. White, and E. Walker. 2013. *Denver Mountain Parks: 100 Years of the Magnificent Dream*. Silverthorne, CO: John Fielder Publishing. [https://coloradoencyclopedia.org/image/100-years-magnificent-dream-denver-mountain-parks].

Fiore, E. 2018. *Morrison History: All About History from Morrison, Colorado*. Morrison, CO: Morrison Historical Society. [https://morrisonhistory.org/people/john-brisben-walker/#:~:text=In%201887%2C%20Walker%20purchased%20the,what%20is%20today%20Regis%20University].

Fisher, C. 2011. Nature in the City: Urban Environmental History and Central Park. *OAH Magazine of History* 25 (4): 27–31.

Fogel, R. 2000. *The Fourth Great Awakening & the Future of Egalitarianism*. Chicago: University of Chicago Press.

Foote, L. 2018. The Refugee Crisis in the American Civil War. *Reviews in American History* 46 (3): 451–457.

Forbath, W. 1989. The Shaping of the American Labor Movement. *Harvard Law Review* 102 (6): 1109–1256.

Forbes, L. 2000. The Legacy of John Ruskin and an Introduction to Unto This Last. *Organization and Environment* 13 (1): 86–88.

Ford, H. 1922. *My Life and Work*. Garden City, NY: Garden City Publishing Co., Inc.

Ford, T. 1999. Understanding Population Growth in the Peri-Urban Region. *International Journal of Population Geography* 5 (4): 297–311.

Fornara, F. and R. Troffa. 2009. Restorative Experiences and Perceived Affective Qualities in Different Built and Natural Urban Places. In *Revitalising Built Environments: Requalifying Old Places for New Uses*, edited by R. J. Lawrence, H. Turgut, and P. Kellett, 1–10. Istanbul: Istanbul Technical University. [https://www.researchgate.net/publication/228327785].

FPC [Forest Park Conservancy]. 2024. Experience Forest Park: America's Premier Urban Forest. *Forest Park Conservancy*. [https://forestparkconservancy.org/forest-park/].

Frey, W. and R. DeVol. 2000. America's Demography in the New Century: Aging Baby Boomers and New Immigrants as Major Players. *Milken Institute*, 8 March.

Fuller, S. M. 1845. *Woman in the Nineteenth Century*. New York: Greeley & McElrath. [https://archive.org/details/womaninnineteent1845full/page/n7/mode/2up].

Gerlach-Spriggs, N., R. E. Kaufman, and S. B. Warner. 1998. *Restorative Gardens: The Healing Landscape*. New Haven: Yale University Press.

Gesler, W. 1992. Therapeutic Landscapes: Medical Issues in Light of the New Cultural Geography. *Social Science & Medicine* 34 (7): 735–746.

Gesler, W. 1996. Lourdes: Healing in a Place of Pilgrimage. *Health & Place* 2: 95–105.

Gesler, W. 2003. *Healing Places*. Lanham: Rowman & Littlefield Publishers, Inc.

Gesler, W. 2018. Therapeutic Landscapes. In *The International Encyclopedia of Anthropology*, edited H. Callan. New York: Wiley & Sons, Inc. [https://doi.org/10.1002/9781118924396.wbiea1422].

Gianfaldoni, S., G. Tchernev, U. Wollina, M. Garzia Roccia, M. Fioranelli, R. Gianfaldoni, and T. Lotti. 2017. History of the Baths and Thermal Medicine. *Open Access Macedonian Journal of Medical Sciences* 5(4): 566–568.

Gibbens, S. 2017. Creepy Photos Show Abandoned American Resort Towns. *National Geographic*, 6 September. [https://www.nationalgeographic.com/photography/article/poconos-catskills-abandoned- resorts-photos-spd].

Gibson, C. 2024. *American Demographic History Chartbook: 1790 to 2010*. [https://demographicchartbook.com/].

Gifford, R. 1987. *The Motivation of Park Users*. Victoria, BC: Optimal Environments.

Gilborn, C. 1981. *Durant: The Fortunes and Woodland Camps of a Family in the Adirondacks*. Sylvan Beach, NY: North Country Books.

Glaser, S. and J. E. Johnston. 1954. *Index of Hospitals and Sanatoria with Tuberculosis Beds in the United States and Territories as of April 1, 1954*. Washington, D.C.: U.S. Government Printing Office.

Glass, D. and J. Singer. 1972. *Urban Stress: Experiments on Noise and Social Stressors*. New York: Academic Press.

Goines, L. and L. Hagler. 2007. Noise Pollution: A Modern Plague. *Southern Medical Journal* 100 (3): 287–294.

Goldenberg, M., E. Hill, and B. Freidt. 2008. Why Individuals Hike the Appalachian Trail: A Qualitative Approach to Benefits. *Journal of Experiential Education* 30 (3): 277–281.

Goodall, R. 2022. The Rise of Wellness Tourism. *The Boar*. [https://theboar.org/2022/01/the-rise-of-wellness-tourism/].

Grathwohl, C. 2024. Oxford Word of the Year 2024. [https://corp.oup.com/word-of-the-year/].

Grineski, S. E., B. Bolin, and V. Agadjanian. 2006. Tuberculosis and Urban Growth: Class, Race and Disease in Early Phoenix, Arizona, USA. *Health and Place* 12: 603–616.

Gugliotta, G. 2012. New Estimate Raises Civil War Death Toll. *New York Times*, 3 April.

Gura, P. F. 2007. *American Transcendentalism: A History*. New York: Hill and Wang.

Gutheim F. and A. J. Lee. 2006. *Worthy of the Nation: Washington, DC, from L'Enfant to the National Capital Planning Commission*. Baltimore: Johns Hopkins University Press.

Hall, P. D. 1984. *The Organization of American Culture, 1700–1900: Private Institutions, Elites, and the Origins of American Nationality*. New York: New York University Press.

Han, K. 2003. A Reliable and Valid Self-Rating Measure of the Restorative Quality of Natural Environments. *Landscape and Urban Planning* 64: 209–232.

Hansmann, R., S. Hug, and K. Seeland. 2007. Restoration and Stress Relief Through Physical Activities in Forests and Parks. *Urban Forestry and Urban Greening* 6: 213–225.

Harner, J. 2021. *Profiting From the Peak: Landscape and Liberty in Colorado Springs*. Louisville: University Press of Colorado.

Harper, E. S. 2019. "The Ladies Merely Breathed Deeply": Women's Invisible Contributions to the Smoky Mountains Hiking Club. *Journal of Appalachian Studies* 25 (2): 143–164.

Harris, D. N., et al. 2025. *The State of the Nation: 2025 Report*. New Orleans: Tulane University. [https://stateofnation.org/assets/stateofnation/downloads/State%20of%20the%20Nation%20Project.pdf].

Hart, T. A. 2012. *When Lungers Came to Tucson: Seeking Recovery and Discovering Tuberculosis as a Social Disease*. Tucson: University of Arizona, Bachelor's Thesis.

Hartig, T. 2011. Issues in Restorative Environments Research: Matters of Measurement. In *Psicologia Ambiental 2011: Entre los Estudios Urbanos y el Analisis de la Sostenibilidad*, edited by B. Fernandez-Ramirez, C. Hidalgo Villodres, C. Salvador Ferrer, and J. Martos Mendez, 41–66. Almeria, Spain: Universidad de Almeria. ISBN: 978-8-4693-9260-7.

Hartig, T. and H. Staats. 2006. The Need for Psychological Restoration as a Determinant of Environmental Preferences. *Journal of Environmental Psychology* 26: 215–226.

Hartig, T., G. Johansson, and C. Kylin. 2003. Residence in the Social Ecology of Stress and Restoration. *Journal of Social Issues* 59: 611–636.

Hartig, T., K. Korpela, G. W. Evans, and T. Garling. 1997. A Measure of Restorative Quality in Environments. *Scandinavian Housing & Planning Research* 14 (1): 175–194.

Hartig, T., R. Mitchell, S. de Vries, and H. Frumkin. 2014. Nature and Health. *Annual Review of Public Health* 35: 207–228.

HC [History Colorado]. 2021. *Denver Mountain Parks*. [https://www.historycolorado.org/denver-mountain-parks].

Hekmat, N., M. Ramazanova, J. Marques, and J. A. Quintela. 2021. Wellness Tourism Experience on the Rise Post COVID: Behavioural Demand Trends and Expectations. In *Planning and Managing the Experience Economy in Tourism*, edited by R. A. Costa, F. Brandao, Z. Breda, and C. Costa, 215–238. Hershey, PA: IGI Global.

Herzog, T. R., C. P. Maguire, and M. B. Nebel. 2003. Assessing the Restorative Components of Environments. *Journal of Environmental Psychology* 23 (1): 159–170.

Hickey, W. 2014. *A Statistical Analysis of the Work of Bob Ross*. Happy Spreadsheets. [https://andyborne.com/math/StorageForFreebies/TinyLibrary/Art/bob-ross.pdf].

Hill, M. B. 2014. *Hot Springs National Park: Images of America*. Charleston: Arcadia Publishing.

Hoby, T. 2014. *Jefferson County Open Space: Enriching Life Master Plan, 2014–2019*. Golden, CO. [https://www.jeffco.us/DocumentCenter/View/9577/Jeffco-Open-Space-2014-2019-Master-Plan?bidId=].

Hodge, H. C. 1877. *Arizona As it Is, Complied from Notes of Travel During the Years 1874, 1875, and 1876*. New York: Hurd and Houghton.

Holson, L. 2019. The Catskills Are Back. Again. And Again. *New York Times*, 21 June. [https://www.nytimes.com/2019/06/21/travel/catskills-history.html].

Hopman, R. J., R. A. Atchley, P. Atchley, and D. Strayer. 2021. How Nature Helps Replenish Our Depleted Cognitive Reserves and Improves Mood by Increasing Activation of the Brain's Default Mode Network. In *Human Capacity in the Attention Economy*, edited by S Lane and P Atchley, 159–187. Washington, D.C.: American Psychological Association. [https://doi.org/10/1037/0000208-008].

Hopman, R. J., S. B. LoTemplio, E. E. Scott, T. L. McKinney, and D. L. Strayer. 2020. Resting-State Posterior Alpha Power Changes with Prolonged Exposure in a Natural Environment. *Cognitive Research: Principles and Implications* 5 (1): 51. [https://doi.org/10.1186/s41235-020-00247-0].

Hountalas, M. G. and S. Silva. 2009. *The San Francisco Cliff House*. Berkeley: Ten Speed Press.

Howat, J. K. 2005. *Frederic Church*. New Haven: Yale University Press.

Hug, S., T. Hartig, R. Hansmann, L. Seeland, and R. Hornung. 2009. Restorative Qualities of Indoor and Outdoor Exercise Settings as Predictors of Exercise Frequency. *Health and Place* 15 (4): 971–980.

Huynh, L. T. M., A. Gasparatos, J. Su, R. D. Lam, E. I. Grant, and K. Fukushi. 2022. Linking the Nonmaterial Dimensions of Human-Nature Relations and Human Well-being Through Cultural Ecosystem Services. *Sciences Advances* 8: 1–21. [https://science.org/doi/10.1126/sciadv.abn8042].

Iddings, L. M. 1896. Life in the Altitudes: The Colorado Health Plateau. *Scribner's Magazine* February: 136–151.

Ikonte, C., H. Prigmore, A. Dawson, and L. Egede. 2020. Trends in Prevalence of Depression and Serious Psychological Distress in United States Immigrant and Non-Immigrant Populations, 2010–2016. *Journal of Affective Disorders* 274: 719–725.

Ilardi, S. 2009. *The Depression Cure: The 6-Step Program to Beat Depression Without Drugs*. Cambridge, MA: Da Capo Press.

Jackson, J.B. 1994. *A Sense of Place, A Sense of Time*. New Haven: Yale University Press.

Jakle, J. 1981. Touring by Automobile in 1932: The American West as Stereotype. *Annals of Tourism Research* 8(4): 534–549.

Jakle, J. and K. Sculle. 2008. *Motoring: The Highway Experience in America*. Athens: University of Georgia Press.

JCOS [Jefferson County Open Space]. 2020*a*. *Jefferson County Open Space: Conservation Greenprint, 2020–2025*. Golden, CO. [https://www.jeffco.us/DocumentCenter/View/22753/Jeffco-Open-Space-Conservation- Greenprint].

JCOS [Jefferson County Open Space]. 2020*b*. *Jeffco Trails Plan*. Golden, CO. [https://www.jeffco.us/DocumentCenter/View/23641/Jeffco-Trails-Plan-Adopted].

Jefferson, T. 1829. *Notes on the State of Virginia*. Boston: Wells and Lilly.

Jensen, C. R. and S. P. Guthrie. 2006. *Outdoor Recreation in America*. Champaign, IL: Human Kinetics.

Jett, S. 1992. An Introduction to Navajo Sacred Places. *Journal of Cultural Geography* 13 (1): 29–39.

Jones, B. M. 1966. A Burden on the Southwest: Migrant Tuberculars in the Nineteenth Century. *Southwestern Social Science Quarterly* 47 (1): 59–67.

Jones, S. 1986. *Workers at Play: A Social and Economic History of Leisure, 1918–1939*. London: Routledge & Kegan Paul.

Kahn-John, M. and M. Koithan. 2015. Living in Health, Harmony, and Beauty: The Dine (Navajo) Hozho Wellness Philosophy. *Global Advances in Health and Medicine* 4 (3): 24–30.

Kaiser, H. 1982. *Great Camps of the Adirondacks*. Boston: David R. Godline.

Kanabus, A. 2020. Sanatorium: From the First to the Last. *TBFacts*, August. [https://tbfacts.org/sanatorium/].

Kandola, A., G. Ashdown-Franks, J. Hendrikse, C. M. Sabiston, and B. Stubbs. 2019. Physical Activity and Depression: Towards Understanding the Antidepressant Mechanisms of Physical Activity. *Neuroscience and Biobehavioral Reviews* 107: 525–539.

Kang, T. 2017. 160 Years of Central Park: A Brief History. *Central Park Conservancy* 1 June. [https://www.centralparknyc.org/articles/central-park-history#:~:text=It%20was%20a%20huge%20success,project's%20original%20%245%20million%20budget].

Kaplan, R. and S. Kaplan. 1989. *The Experience of Nature: A Psychological Perspective*. New York: Cambridge University Press.

Kaplan, S. 1995. The Restorative Benefits of Nature: Toward an Integrative Framework. *Journal of Environmental Psychology* 15 (3): 169–182.

Katsingris, P. 2020. *The Nielsen Total Audience Report, August 2020: Special Work from Home Edition*. The Nielsen Company. [https://www.nielsen.com/us/en/insights/report/2020/the-nielsen-total-audience-report-august-2020/].

Keers, R. Y. 1980. Two Forgotten Pioneers, James Carson and George Bodington. *Thorax* 35 (7): 483–489.

Kellert, S., J. Heerwagen, and M. Mador. 2008. *Biophilic Design: The Theory, Science, and Practice of Bringing Buildings to Life*. Bridgewater, NJ: John Wiley & Sons.

Kemmis, D. 1990. *Community and the Politics of Place*. Norman: University of Oklahoma Press.

Kennedy, D. 1975. Overview: The Progressive Era. *The Historian (Kingston)* 37 (3): 453–468.

Kennedy, D. 2018. *Resident Survey, 2018: A Report to Jefferson County Open Space*. Denver: Corona Insights. [https://www.jeffco.us/DocumentCenter/View/16575/Jeffco-Open-Space-2018-Resident- Survey-Results].

Kennedy, L. W. 1992. *Planning the City Upon a Hill: Boston Since 1630*. Amherst: University of Massachusetts Press.

Khodaei, M., A. Noorbala, Z. Parsian, S. Targhi, F. Emadi, F. Alijaniha, M. Naseri, and A. Zargaran. 2017. Avicenna (980–1032 CE): The Pioneer in Treatment of Depression. *Transylvanian Review* 24 (17): 4377–4389.

Kilbourne, F. W. 1916. *Chronicles of the White Mountains*. Boston: Houghton Mifflin Company.

Kinnealey, M. and M. Fuiek. 1999. The Relationship Between Sensory Defensiveness, Anxiety, Depression and Perception of Pain in Adults. *Occupational Therapy International* 6 (3): 195–206.

Korpela, K. and T. Hartig. 1996. Restorative Qualities of Favorite Places. *Journal of Environmental Psychology* 16: 221–233.

Korpela, K., M. Ylen, L. Tyrvainen, and H. Silvennoinen. 2008. Determinants of Restorative Experiences in Everyday Favorite Places. *Health & Place* 14: 636–652.

Korpela, K., T. Hartig, F. Kaiser, and U. Fuhrer. 2001. Restorative Experience and Self- Regulation in Favorite Places. *Environment and Behavior* 33 (4): 572–589.

Kosanic, A. and J. Petzold. 2020. A Systematic Review of Cultural Ecosystem Services and Human Wellbeing. *Ecosystem Services* 45. [https://doi.org/10.1016/j.ecoser.2020.101168].

Kowalski, A. and R. H. Ross. 1993. *Bob Ross' New Joy of Painting: A Collection of His Favorites*. New York: William Morrow.

Kramer, D. 2010. The Effects of Psychological Torture. *Berkeley Law—International Human Rights Law Clinic*. [https://www.law.berkeley.edu/experiential/clinics/international-human-rights-law-clinic/do-no-harm-intelligence-ethics-health-professionals-and-the-torture-debate/effects-of-psychological-torture/].

Kranowitz, C. S. 2005. *The Out-Of-Sync Child: Recognizing and Coping with Sensory Processing Disorder*. New York: Penguin.

Kuo, F. E. and A. F. Taylor. 2004. A Potential Natural Treatment for Attention- Deficit/Hyperactivity Disorder: Evidence from a National Study. *American Journal of Public Health* 94 (9): 1580–1597.

LandScope. 2021. Open Space 101. *LandScope America*. [http://www.landscope.org/explore/open_space_101/].

Larson, E. K., S. Earl, E. M. Hagen, R. Hale, H. Hartnett, M. McCrackin, M. McHale, and N. B. Grimm. 2013. Beyond Restoration and into Design: Hydrologic Alterations in Aridland Cities. In *Resilience in Ecology and Urban Design*, edited by S. T. A. Pickett, M. L. Cadenasso, and Brian McGrath, 183–210. New York: Springer.

Laumann, K., T. Garling, and K. Stormark. 2001. Rating Scale Measures of Restorative Components of Environments. *Journal of Environmental Psychology* 21: 31–44.

Laumann, K., T. Garling, and K. Stormark. 2003. Selective Attention and Heart Rate Responses to Natural and Urban Environments. *Journal of Environmental Psychology* 23: 125–134.

Lawless, L., C. Loughlin, and L. Meier. 2008. *The Master List of Design Projects of the Olmsted Firm, 1857–1979*. Washington, D.C.: National Association for Olmsted Parks.

Laws, J. 2009. Reworking Therapeutic Landscapes: The Spatiality of an 'Alternative' Self-Help Group. *Social Science and Medicine* 69 (10): 1827–1833.

Lederbogen, F., et al. 2011. City Living and Urban Upbringing Affect Neural Social Stress Processing in Humans. *Nature* 474 (6): 498–501.

Lehto, X. 2012. Assessing the Perceived Restorative Qualities of Vacation Destinations. *Journal of Travel Research* 52 (3): 325–339.

Lenger, F. 1991. Beyond Exceptionalism: Notes on the Artisanal Phase of the Labour Movement in France, England, Germany and the United States. *International Review of Social History* 36 (1): 1–23.

Leonard, S. and T. Noel. 1990. *Denver: Mining Camp to Metropolis*. Niwot: University Press of Colorado.

Leonhardt, D. 2022. On the Phone, Alone. *New York Times*, 10 May.

Leonhardt, D. 2023. The Phone in the Room. *New York Times*, 27 February.

Levitin, D. J. 2015. *The Organized Mind: Thinking Straight in the Age of Information Overload*. New York: Plume.

Lewicka, M. 2011. Place Attachment: How Far Have We Come in the Last 40 Years? *Journal of Environmental Psychology* 31: 207–230.

Liss, M., J. Mailloux, and M. J. Erchull. 2008. The Relationships Between Sensory Processing Sensitivity, Alexithymia, Autism, Depression, and Anxiety. *Personality and Individual Differences* 45 (3): 255–259.

Livingston, M., N. Bailey, and A. Kearns. 2008. *People's Attachment to Place—The Influence of Neighborhood Deprivation*. York, UK: The Joseph Rountree Foundation.

Louv, R. 2005. *Last Child in the Woods: Saving Our Children from Nature-Deficit Disorder*. Chapel Hill: Algonquin Books of Chapel Hill.

Low, S. M. and I. Altman. 1992. Place Attachment: A Conceptual Inquiry. In *Place Attachment*, edited by I. Altman and S. M. Low, 1–12. New York: Plenum Press.

Luce, C. 2014. *The White Plague in the City of Angels*. Los Angeles: Scalar. [https://scalar.usc.edu/hc/tuberculosis-exhibit/index].

MacDougall, H. 1990. *James Fenimore Cooper: Pioneer of the Environmental Movement*. James Fenimore Cooper Society. [https://jfcoopersociety.org/articles/informal/hugh-environment.html].

MacKaye, B. 1921. An Appalachian Trail: A Project in Regional Planning. *Journal of American Institute of Architects* 9: 3–8.

MacKerron, G. and S. Mourato. 2013. Happiness is Greater in Natural Environments. *Global Environmental Change* 23: 992–1000.

Maller, C., C. Henderson-Wilson, and M. Townsend. 2009. Rediscovering Nature in Everyday Settings: Or How to Create Healthy Environments and Healthy People. *EcoHealth* 6 (4): 553–556.

Maller, C., M. Townsend, A. Pryor, P. Brown, and L. St. Leger. 2005. Healthy Nature Healthy People: 'Contact with Nature' as an Upstream Health Promotion Intervention for Populations. *Health Promotion International* 21 (1): 45–54.

Manzo, L. C. and P. Devine-Wright. 2014. *Place Attachment: Advances in Theory, Methods, and Applications*. London: Routledge.

Marcus, C. C. and N. A. Sachs. 2014. *Therapeutic Landscapes: An Evidence-Based Approach to Designing Healing Gardens and Restorative Outdoor Spaces*. Hoboken: John Wiley & Sons.

Marra, S. 2021. The Work Ahead. *Appalachian Trail Conservancy*, 15 October. [https://appalachiantrail.org/official-blog/the-work-ahead/].

Marwick, A. 1968. The Impact of the First World War on British Society. *Journal of Contemporary History* 3 (1): 51–63.

Mattila, O., A. Korhonen, E. Poyry, K. Hauru, J. Holopainen, and P. Parvinen. 2020. Restoration in a Virtual Reality Forest Environment. *Computers in Human Behavior* 107: 106295.

McKay, D. R. 1979. A History of the Nordrach Ranch: Colorado's First Sanatorium of the Open Air. *Colorado Magazine* 56: 179–196.

McKnight-Nichols, C. and N. C. Unger. 2017. Introduction: Gilded Excesses, Multiple Progressivisms. In *A Companion to the Gilded Age and Progressive Era,* edited by C. McKnight-Nichols and N. C. Unger, 1–4. West Sussex: John Wiley & Sons, Inc.

McLean, D. D. and A. R. Hurd. 2015. *Kraus' Recreation and Leisure in Modern Society, Tenth Edition*. Burlington, MA: Jones & Bartlett Learning.

McMichael, A., R. Scholes, M. Hefny, E. Pereira, C. Palm, and S. Foale. 2005. Linking Ecosystem Services and Human Well-being. In *Ecosystems and Human Well-being: Multiscale Assessment*, edited by C. Capistrano, M. J. Lee, C. Raudsepp-Hearne, and K. Samper, 43–60. Washington, D.C.: Island Press.

Melder, F. E. 1960. The "Tin Lizzie's" Golden Anniversary. *American Quarterly* 12 (4): 466–481.

Meyer, J. 2021. Good News, Hikers: Denver Mountain Parks Growing for First Time Since 1939. *The Denver Post,* 11 February. [https://theknow-old.denverpost.com/2021/02/11/denver-mountain-parks-golden-gate-state-park-bigger/253137/].

Mnassar, S. 2015. Competing Environmental Ethics in Cooper's 'The Pioneers'. *Advances in Language and Literary Studies* 6 (2): 78–86.

Mossabir, R., C. Milligan, and K. Froggatt. 2021. Therapeutic Landscape Experiences of Everyday Geographies Within the Wider Community: A Scoping Review. *Social Science & Medicine*. [doi.org/101016/jsocscimed.2021.113980].

Muir, J. 1898. The Wild Parks and Forest Reservations of the West. *The Atlantic Monthly* 81: 15–28.

Muir, J. 1901. *Our National Parks*. Boston: Houghton Mifflin and Company. Muir, J. 1912. *The Yosemite*. New York: The Century Co.

Murray, W. H. H. 1869. *Adventures in the Wilderness; or, Camp-Life in the Adirondacks*. Boston: Fields, Osgood, & Co.

Myers, K. 1988. *The Catskills: Painters, Writers, and Tourists in the Mountains (1820–1895)*. Yonkers: Hudson River Museum of Westchester.

Myerson, J. 2000. *Transcendentalism: A Reader*. Oxford: Oxford University Press.

NAMI [National Alliance on Mental Illness]. 2020. *Mental Health by the Numbers*. [https://www.nami.org/mhstats].

Nash, R. F. 1989. *The Rights of Nature: A History of Environmental Ethics*. Madison: University of Wisconsin Press.

Negrin, F., E. Hernandez-Fernaud, S. Hess, and B. Hernandez. 2017. Discrimination of Urban Spaces with Different Level of Restorativeness Based on the Original and on a Shorter Version of Hartig et al.'s Perceived Restorativeness Scale. *Frontiers in Psychology* 9 October. [https://www.frontiersin.org/articles/10.3389/fpsyg.2017.01735/full].

Nemade, R. and K. Patricelli. 2020. Historical Understanding of Depression. *SEABHS*. [https://www.seabhs.org/poc/view_doc.php?type=doc&id=12995&cn=5].

Neufeld, R. 2019. Visiting Our Past: Asheville Was Flush With a "Magic Mountain" High. *Asheville Citizen Times*, 7 April. [https://www.citizen- times.com/story/news/2019/04/07/visiting-our-past-asheville-flush-magic-mountain- high/3351019002/].

Newcomb, F. 1967. *Navaho Folk Tales*. Albuquerque: University of New Mexico Press.

Nordh, H., T. Hartig, C. Hagerhall, and G. Fry. 2009. Components of Small Urban Parks that Predict the Possibility for Restoration. *Urban Forestry and Urban Greening* 8: 225–235.

Nota, G., R. Marian, G. Callegari, R. Berto, and G. Barbiero. 2017. When Biophilic Design Meets Restorative Architecture: The Strambinello Project. *Visions for Sustainability* 8: 46–58.

Novak, B. 1980. *Nature and Culture: American Landscape Painting, 1825–1875*. New York: Oxford University Press.

Nowak, D. J. 2002. *The Effects of Urban Trees on Air Quality*. Syracuse: USDA Forest Service. [https://www.nrs.fs.fed.us/units/urban/local-resources/downloads/Tree_Air_Qual.pdf].

NPF [National Park Foundation]. 2021. *The Hike of a Lifetime: Appalachian National Scenic Trail*. Washington, D.C.: National Park Foundation. [https://www.nationalparks.org/connect/explore-parks/appalachian-national-scenic-trail].

NPS [National Park Service]. 2020. *Hot Springs National Park Arkansas*. Washington, D.C.: U.S. Government Printing Office, U.S. Department of the Interior.

Nye, N. C. 2020. Hiking in America: Historical Context. *Forest History Society*. [https://foresthistory.org/research-explore/us-forest-service-history/policy-and-law/recreation-u-s-forest-service/hiking-in-america/].

OF. 2021. 2021 Outdoor Participation Trends Report. Boulder: *Outdoor Foundation*. 22 June. [https://outdoorindustry.org/wp-content/uploads/2015/03/2021-Outdoor-Participation-Trends-Report.pdf].

Olmsted, F. L. and L. W. Roper. 1952. The Yosemite Valley and the Mariposa Big Trees: A Preliminary Report (1865). *Landscape Architecture Magazine* 43 (1): 12–25.

Onion, A., M. Sullivan, M. Mullen, and C. Zapata. 2010. Model T. *History.com/editors*, 26 April. [https://www.history.com/articles/model-t].

Oplinger, C. and R. Halma. 2006. *The Poconos: An Illustrated Natural History Guide*. New Brunswick: Rutgers University Press.

Ortiz-Ospina, E. 2019. The Rise of Social Media. *OurWorldInData.org*. [https://ourworldindata.org/rise-of-social-media].

Packer, B. L. 2007. *The Transcendentalists*. Athens: University of Georgia Press.

Packer, J. and N. Bond. 2010. Museums as Restorative Environments. *Curator* 53 (4): 421–436.

Paige, J. C. and L. S. Harrison. 1988. *Out of the Vapors: A Social and Architectural History of Bathhouse Row, Hot Springs National Park, Arkansas*. Washington, D.C.: U.S. National Park Service.

Palomino, M., T. Taylor, A. Goker, J. Isaacs, and S. Warber. 2016. The Online Dissemination of Nature–Health Concepts: Lessons from Sentiment Analysis of Social Media Relating to "Nature-Deficit Disorder". *International Journal of Environmental Research and Public Health* 13 (1): 142–165.

Pals, R., L Steg, F. Siero, and K. Van der Zee. 2009. Development of the PRCQ: A Measure of Perceived Restorative Characteristics of Zoo Attractions. *Journal of Environmental Psychology* 29: 441–449.

Payne, A. and D. Hurt. 2024. The Making of an American Cultural Icon: Postcard Imagery and Place Promotion Along Route 66. *Material Culture* 56 (1): 31–51.

Perrottet, T. 2013. Where Was the Birthplace of the American Vacation? *Smithsonian Magazine*, April. [https://www.smithsonianmag.com/travel/where-was-the-birthplace-of-the-american-vacation-5520155/].

Peschardt, K. and U. Stigsdotter. 2013. Associations Between Park Characteristics and Perceived Restorativeness of Small Public Urban Green Spaces. *Landscape and Urban Planning* 112 (1): 26–39.

Peterson, T. R. 1991. Telling the Farmers' Story: Competing Responses to Soil Conservation Rhetoric. *Quarterly Journal of Speech* 77 (3): 289–308.

Pratt, L. A. and D. J. Brody. 2008. Depression in the United States Household Population, 2005–2006. *National Center for Health Statistics, Publication No. 2008–1209, U.S.*

Department of Health and Human Services. [https://www.cdc.gov/nchs/data/databriefs/db07.pdf].

Quinn, J. and C. Helmstetter. 2019. How Often Do Americans Spend Free Time in Nature? *APM Research Lab*, 15 July. [https://www.apmresearchlab.org/nature].

Reese, R., S. Hadeed, H. Craig, A. Beyer, and M. Gosling. 2019. EcoWellness: Integrating the Natural World into Wilderness Therapy Settings with Intentionality. *Journal of Adventure Education and Outdoor Learning* 19 (3): 202–215.

Reese, R. and J. Myers. 2012. EcoWellness: The Missing Factor in Holistic Wellness Models. *Journal of Counseling and Development* 9 (4): 400–406.

Rex-Atzet, W. 2011. *Denver's Mountain Playground: The Denver Mountain Parks, The City Beautiful, and the Rise of Modern Wilderness Recreation in Colorado, 1900–1940*. Ph.D. diss. University of Colorado. [https://scholar.colorado.edu/concern/graduate_thesis_or_dissertations/w9505052n].

Rex-Atzet, W. 2020. Denver Mountain Parks. *Colorado Encyclopedia*, 14 February. [https://coloradoencyclopedia.org/article/denver-mountain-parks].

Rice-Oxley, M. 2019. Mental Illness: Is There Really a Global Epidemic? *The Guardian*. 3 June. [https://www.theguardian.com/society/2019/jun/03/mental-illness-is-there-really-a-global-epidemic].

Richardson, H. C. 2017. Reconstructing the Gilded Age and Progressive Era. In *A Companion to the Gilded Age and Progressive Era,* edited by C. McKnight Nichols and N. C. Unger, 7–20. West Sussex: John Wiley & Sons, Inc.

Richardson, R. 1995. *Emerson: The Mind on Fire*. Berkeley: University of California Press.

Richtel, M. 2010. Growing Up Digital, Wired for Distraction. *New York Times*. 21 November. [https://www.nytimes.com/2010/11/21/technology/21brain.html?searchResultPosition=2].

Riis, J. A. 1890. *How the Other Half Lives: Studies Among the Tenements of New York*. New York: Charles Scribner's Sons. [https://www.gutenberg.org/files/45502/45502-h/45502-h.htm].

Roe, J. and L. McCay. 2021. *Restorative Cities: Urban Design for Mental Health and Wellbeing*. London: Bloomsbury Visual Arts.

Rosenbaum, M. and I. Wong. 2015. When Gambling Is Healthy: The Restorative Potential of Casinos. *Journal of Services Marketing* 29 (6–7): 622–633.

Rosenbaum, M., L. Otalora, and G. Contreras Ramirez. 2016. The Restorative Potential of Shopping Malls. *Journal of Retailing and Consumer Services* 31 (2): 157–165.

Rosenzweig, R. and E. Blackmar. 1992. *The Park and the People: A History of Central Park*. Ithaca: Cornell University Press.

Rothman, S. M. 1994. *Living in the Shadow of Death: Tuberculosis and the Social Experience of Illness in American History*. New York: Harper Collins Publishers.

Rowley, R. 2020. Antecedent Landscapes and Las Vegas Casinos: Exploring Place Through a Referential Perspective. *Material Culture* 52 (1): 1–25.

Rowthorn, A. 2012. *The Wisdom of John Muir: 100+ Selections from the Letters, Journals, and Essays of the Great Naturalist*. Birmingham: Wilderness Press.

Rubissow, A. 1993. *Cliff House and Lands End: San Francisco's Seaside Retreat*. San Francisco: Golden Gate National Park Association.

Rudd-Jones, N. 2015. A Brief History of Urban Green Spaces. *Urban Rambles* 28 December. [https://urbanrambles.org/background/a-brief-history-of-rus-in-urbe-1307].

Ruggles, S. 2015. Patriarchy, Power, and Pay: The Transformation of American Families, 1800–2015. *Demography* 52(6): 1797–1823.

Ruskin, J. 1903. *Modern Painters: Volume II*. London: George Allen. [https://wayback.archive-it.org/all/20170418201223/http://www.lancaster.ac.uk/depts/ruskinlib/Modern%20Painters#.pdf].

Ruskin, J. A. 1990. Thomas Cole and the White Mountains: The Picturesque, the Sublime, and the Magnificent. *Bulletin of the Detroit Institute of Arts* 66 (1): 18–25.

Ryan, C., W. Browning, J. Clancy, S. Andrews, and N. Kallianpurkar. 2014. Biophilic Design Patterns: Emerging Nature-Based Parameters for Health and Well-Being in the Built Environment. *International Journal of Architectural Research* 8 (2): 62–76.

Ryan, M., S. R. Lawson, A. M. Larkin, S. J. Roberts, and D. Pettebone. 2020. Engaging Minority Communities in Local National Park Units Through Culturally Competent Focus Groups. *Journal of Park and Recreation Administration* 38 (1): 67–87.

Rybczynski, W. 1999. *A Clearing in the Distance: Frederick Law Olmsted and America in the Nineteenth Century*. New York: Scribner.

Sacks, K. S. 2003. *Understanding Emerson: The American Scholar and his Struggle for Self-Reliance*. Princeton: Princeton University Press.

SAMHSA [Substance Abuse and Mental Health Services Administration]. 2024. *Key Substance Use and Mental Health Indicators in the United States: Results from the 2018 National Survey on Drug Use and Health* (Department of Health and Human Services Publication No. PEP19–5068, NSDUH Series H-54). Rockville, MD: Center for Behavioral Health Statistics and Quality, SAMHSA. [https://www.samhsa.gov/data/].

Scannell, L. and R. Gifford. 2010. Defining Place Attachment: A Tripartite Organizing Framework. *Journal of Environmental Psychology* 30: 1–10.

Schebella, M. F., D. Weber, K. Lindsey, and C. B. Daniels. 2017. For the Love of Nature: Exploring the Importance of Species Diversity and Micro-Variables Associated with Favorite Outdoor Places. *Frontiers in Psychology* 8: 2094. [https://doi.org/10.3389/fpsyg.2017.02094].

Scheydt, S., M. M. Staub, F. Frauenfelder, G. H. Nielsen, J. Behrens, and I Needham. 2017. Review Article: Sensory Overload: A Concept Analysis. *International Journal of Mental Health Nursing* 26: 110–120.

Schimelpfening, N. and A. Morin. 2020. The History of Depression: Accounts, Treatments, and Beliefs Through the Ages. *Verywellmind*. 25 February. [https://www.verywellmind.com/who-discovered-depression-1066770].

Schlett, J. 2015. *A Not Too Greatly Changed Eden: The Story of the Philosophers' Camp in the Adirondacks*. Ithaca: Cornell University Press.

Schmalz, D. L., J. C. Hallo, S. F. Griffin, M. Kusch, and M. Arce. 2013. Development of a Healthy Parks Healthy People Strategic Action Plan for Hot Springs National Park. *Park Science* 30 (2): 37–43.

Schmidt, S. 2008. The Evolving Relationship Between Open Space Preservation and Local Planning Practice. *Journal of Planning History* 7 (2): 91–112.

Scopelliti, M., G. Carrus, and M. Bonaiuto. 2019. Is it Really Nature That Restores People? A Comparison with Historical Sites With High Restorative Potential. *Frontiers in Psychology* 9: 02742. [https://www.frontiersin.org/articles/10.3389/fpsyg.2018.02742/full].

Scopelliti, M. and M. V. Giuliani. 2004. Choosing Restorative Environments Across the Lifespan: A Matter of Place Experience. *Journal of Environmental Psychology* 24: 423–437.

Seagren, K. 2021. *Why I Hike*. Appalachian Trail Conservancy. [https://appalachiantrail.org/news-events/why-i-hike/kenny-seagren/].

Seamon, D. 2014. Place Attachment and Phenomenology: The Synergistic Dynamism of Place. In *Place Attachment: Advances in Theory, Methods, and Applications,* edited by L. Manzo and P. Devine-Wright, 11–22. London: Routledge.

Seamon, D. and A. Lundberg. 2017. Humanistic Geography. In *The International Encyclopedia of Geography: People, the Earth, Environment and Technology*, ed. by D. Richardson, N. Castree, M. Goodchild, A. Kobayashi, W. Liu, and R. Marston, 1–11. Bridgewater, NY: John Wiley & Sons, Ltd.

Seo, H. 2023. America is Getting Lonelier and More Indoorsy. *The Atlantic*, 13 November.

Shivers, J. and L. deLisle. 1997. *The Story of Leisure: Context, Concepts, and Current Controversy*. Champaign, IL: Human Kinetics.

Shrieves, L. 1990. Bob Ross Uses His Brush to Spread Paint and Joy. *Orlando Sentinel*, 7 July. [http://articles.orlandosentinel.com/1990-07-07/lifestyle/9007060122_1_bob-ross-joy-of-painting-pbs].

Sinclair, Mick. 2004. *San Francisco: A Cultural and Literary History*. Oxford: Signal Books.

Smith, C. 2009. Taming the Savage City: One Hundred Years Later, Daniel Burnham's Plan of Chicago Still Inspires. *Humanities* 30(5): 1–15. [https://www.neh.gov/humanities/2009/septemberoctober/feature/taming-the-savage-city].

Smith, J. R. 2005. *San Francisco's Lost Landmarks*. Sanger, CA: Word Dancer Press.

Smith, J. S. 2018. *Explorations in Place Attachment*. London: Routledge.

Song, C., H. Ikei, and Y. Miyazaki. 2016. Physiological Effects of Nature Therapy: A Review of Research in Japan. *International Journal of Environmental Research and Public Health* 13: 78–95.

Souter-Brown, G. 2014. *Landscape and Urban Design for Health and Well Being: Using Healing, Sensory and Therapeutic Gardens*. London: Routledge.

Sparling, P., N. Owen, E. Lambert, and W. Haskell. 2000. Promoting Physical Activity: The New Imperative for Public Health. *Health Education Research* 15 (3): 367–376.

Spaulding, J. H. 1858. *Guide and Historical Relics of the White Mountains*. Mt. Washington: J. H. Spaulding.

Squeri, L. 2002. *Better in the Poconos: The Story of Pennsylvania's Vacationland*. University Park, PA: Pennsylvania State University Press.

Staats, H., A. Kieviet, and T. Hartig. 2003. When to Recover from Attentional Fatigue: An Expectancy-Value Analysis of Environmental Preference. *Journal of Environmental Psychology* 23: 147–157.

Stanley, B. W., B. L. Stark, K. L. Johnston, and M. E. Smith. 2012. Urban Open Spaces in Historical Perspective: A Transdisciplinary Typology and Analysis. *Urban Geography* 33 (8): 1089–1117.

STAR [STAR Institute]. 2023. SPD [Sensory Processing Disorder] Latest Research Findings. *STAR Institute*. [https://sensoryhealth.org/basic/latest-research-findings].

Statista. 2022. *City Parks in the U.S. by Annual Visitorship in 2020*. [https://www.statista.com/statistics/190057/number-of-visitors-to-city-parks-in-the-us-2009/].

Stephenson, A. B. 1989. Secrets of the Model T. *American Heritage* 40 (5): 73–77.

Stewart, F. 1995. *A Natural History of Nature Writing*. Washington, D.C.: Island Press.

Stewart-Pollack, J. 2006. Biophilic Design for the First Optimum Performance Home. *Ultimate Home Design* 4: 36–41.

Stillman, W. J. 1901. *The Autobiography of a Journalist*. London: Grant Richards.

Stout, C. K. 1997. *A Consumptives' Refuge: Colorado and Tuberculosis*. Ph.D. diss. George Washington University.

Stradling, D. 2007. *Making Mountains: New York City and the Catskills*. Seattle: University of Washington Press.

Strochlic, N. 2022. Borscht Belt Revisited. *National Geographic* (August): 28–30.

Subiza-Perez, M., L. Vozmediano, and C. San Juan. 2020. Welcome to Your Plaza: Assessing the Restorative Potential of Urban Squares Through Survey and Objective Evaluation Methods. *Cities* 100: 102461.

Sullivan, J. 2021. *Why I Hike*. Appalachian Trail Conservancy. [https://appalachiantrail.org/news-events/why-i-hike/janene-sullivan/].

Summers, J. K. and D. N. Vivian. 2018. Ecotherapy—A Forgotten Ecosystem Service: A Review. *Frontiers in Psychology* 9 (8): 1–13.

Takano, T., K. Nakamura, and M. Watanabe. 2002. Urban Residential Environments and Senior Citizens' Longevity in Megacity Areas: The Importance of Walkable Green Spaces. *Journal of Epidemiology and Community Health* 56: 913–918.

Tarbell, I. 1902. Miss Tarbell's History of the Standard Oil Company. *McClure's Magazine* 19 (6): 589–592.

Teale, E. W. 1954. *The Wilderness World of John Muir*. Boston: Houghton Mifflin Co.

Thoreau, H. D. 1854. *Walden: or, Life in the Woods*. Boston: Ticknor and Fields.

Thoreau, H. D. 1862. Walking. *Atlantic Monthly* 9 (56): 657–674.

Tolles, Jr., B. F. 1998. *The Grand Resort Hotels of the White Mountains: A Vanishing Architectural Legacy*. Boston: David R. Godine.

Townsend, M., C. Henderson-Wilson, H. Ramkissoon, and R. Weerasuriya. 2018. Therapeutic Landscapes, Restorative Environments, Place Attachment, and Well-being. In *Oxford Textbook of Nature and Public Health: The Role of Nature in Improving the Health of a Population*, edited by M. van den Bosch and W. Bird, 57–62. Oxford: Oxford University Press.

Tuan, Y. 1974. *Topophilia: A Study of Environmental Perception, Attitudes, and Values*. Englewood Cliffs, NJ: Prentice-Hall Inc.

Tuan, Y. 1977. *Space and Place: The Perspective of Experience*. Minneapolis: University of Minnesota Press.

Turner, W., T. Nakamura, and M. Dinetti. 2004. Global Urbanization and the Separation of Humans from Nature. *BioScience* 54 (6): 585–590.

Twain, M. 1864. A Trip to the Cliff House. *San Francisco Daily Morning Call*, 25 June. [http://www.twainquotes.com/callindex.html].

Twain, M. and C. D. Warner. 1873. *The Gilded Age: A Tale of Today*. New York: American Publishing Company.

Tyson, M. 1998. *The Healing Landscape: Therapeutic Outdoor Environments*. New York: McGraw-Hill.

Ulrich, R. S. 1984. View Through a Window May Influence Recovery from Surgery. *Science* 224(4): 420–421.

UNESCO [United Nations Educational, Scientific and Cultural Organization]. 2021. *The Great Spa Towns of Europe*. New York: United Nations Printing Office. [https://whc.unesco.org/en/list/1613/].

U.S. Census. 2021. *Measuring Household Experiences During the Coronavirus Pandemic: Household Pulse Survey-Phase 3.1*. Washington, D.C.: U.S. Department of Commerce. [https://www.census.gov/data/experimental-data-products/household-pulse-survey.html].

U.S. Census. 2022. *Manhattan Borough, New York County, New York*. Washington, D.C.: U.S. Bureau of the Census. [https://www.census.gov/search-results.html?searchType=web&cssp=SERP&q=Manhattan%20borough,%20New%20York%20County,%20New%20York].

USDOT [United States Department of Transportation]. 2022. *History of the Federal Highway Administration*. Washington, D.C. [https://highways.dot.gov/federal-lands/about/history].

Van Buren, A. 2016. 12 Secrets of New York's Central Park: Lean Some Little-Known Facts about this NYC Landmark. *Smithsonian*, 27 January. [https://www.smithsonianmag.com/travel/12-secrets-new-yorks-central-park-180957937/].

Van den Berg, A., A. Jorgensen, and E. Wilson. 2014. Evaluating Restoration in Urban Green Spaces: Does Setting Type Make a Difference? *Landscape and Urban Planning* 127: 173–181.

Visit KC. 2022. *Super Cities: Comparing Kansas City and Tampa Bay*. Kansas City: Kansas City Tourism Office. [https://www.visitkc.com/super-cities-comparing-kansas-city-and-tampa-bay].

Voss, K. and R. Sherman. 2000. Breaking the Iron Law of Oligarchy: Union Revitalization in the American Labor Movement. *American Journal of Sociology* 106 (2): 303–349.

Walker, C. 2004. *The Public Value of Urban Parks*. Washington, D.C.: The Urban Institute. [https://www.urban.org/sites/default/files/publication/57651/311011-The-Public-Value-of-Urban-Parks.PDF].

Wallis, M. 2001. *Route 66: The Mother Road (75th Anniversary Edition)*. New York: St. Martin's Griffin.

Walls, L. D. 2017. *Henry David Thoreau: A Life*. Chicago: University of Chicago Press.

Wang, C., L. Geng, and J. D. Rodriguez-Casallas. 2023. The Role of Nature-Deficit Disorder in the Associations Between Mobile Phone Overuse and Well-being and Mindfulness. *Current Psychology* 42 (2): 894–905.

Weber, J. and S. Sultana. 2013. Why Do So Few Minority People Visit National Parks?: Visitation and the Accessibility of "America's Best Idea". *Annals of the Association of American Geographers* 103 (3): 437–464.

Weeks, J. 1883. *Report on the Statistics of Wages in Manufacturing Industries, 1880*. Washington, D.C.: United States, Department of Interior, Census Office.

Weingroff, R. F. 1996. Federal-Aid Highway Act of 1956: Creating the Interstate System. *Public Roads, USDOT* 60(1). [https://highways.dot.gov/public-roads/summer-1996/federal-aid-highway-act-1956-creating-interstate-system#:~:text=Fallon%20introduced%20a%20revised%20bill,90%20percent%20or%20%2424.8%20billion].

Weiss, T. 2004. Tourism in America Before World War II. *Journal of Economic History* 64 (2): 289–327.

Wetmore, C. H. and L. Steffens. 1902. Tweed Days in St. Louis. *McClure's Magazine* 19 (10): 577–586.

Whaples, R. 2001. Hours of Work in U.S. History. *EH.net Encyclopedia*. [http://eh.net/encyclopedia/hours-of-work-in-u-s-history/].

White, E. M., J. M. Bowker, A. E. Askew, L. L. Langner, J. R. Arnold, and D. B. K. English. 2016. *Federal Outdoor Recreation Trends: Effects on Economic Opportunities*. General Technical Report PNW-GTR-945. Washington, D.C.: U.S. Department of Agriculture.

White, R. 2017. *The Republic for Which it Stands: The United States During Reconstruction and the Gilded Age, 1865–1896*. New York: Oxford University Press.

WHO [World Health Organization]. 2019. *Mental Disorders Fact Sheets*. 28 November. Geneva: WHO Document Production Services. [https://www.who.int/en/news-room/fact-sheets/detail/mental-disorders].

WHO [World Health Organization]. 2021. *Comprehensive Mental Health Action Plan, 2013–2020*. Geneva: WHO Document Production Services. License: CC BY-NC-SA 3.0 IGO.

WHO [World Health Organization]. 2022. *Mental Disorders Fact Sheets*. 8 June. Geneva: WHO Document Production Services. [https://www.who.int/en/news-room/fact-sheets/detail/mental-disorders].

Willey, B. G. and F. Thompson. 1870. *History of the White Mountains*. New York: Hurd and Houghton.

Williams, A. (ed). 1999. *Therapeutic Landscapes: The Dynamic Between Place and Wellness*. Lanham: University Press of America, Inc.

Williams, A. (ed). 2007. *Therapeutic Landscapes*. London: Routledge.

Williams, A. 2009. Therapeutic Landscapes as Health Promoting Places. In *A Companion to Health and Medical Geography*, edited by T. Brown, S. McLafferty, and G. Moon, 205–223. Hoboken: John Wiley & Sons.

Williams, F. 2016. This is Your Brain on Nature: When We Get Closer to Nature—Be in Untouched Wilderness or a Backyard Tree—We Do Our Overstressed Brains a Favor. *National Geographic* 229 (1): 48–67.

Williams, F. 2017. *The Nature Fix: Why Nature Makes Us Happier, Healthier, and More Creative*. New York: W.W. Norton & Co.

Wilson, A. and G. Dennison. 1995. *Navajo Place Names*. Guilford, CT: Jeffrey Norton Publishers.

Wilson, E. 1984. *Biophilia: The Human Bond with Other Species*. Cambridge: Harvard University Press.

Winter, P. L., S. Selin, L. Cerveny, and K. Bricker. 2020. Outdoor Recreation, Nature-Based Tourism, and Sustainability. *Sustainability* 12 (1): 81–93.

Witte, M. 2017. *Happy Little Accidents: The Wit and Wisdom of Bob Ross*. Philadelphia: Running Press Book Publishers.

Witters, D. 2023. *U.S. Depression Rates Reach New High*. Washington, D.C.: Gallup, Inc. [https://news.gallup.com/poll/505745/depression-rates-reach-new-highs.aspx#:~:text =In%202023%2C%2029.0%25%20of%20Americans,17.8%25%20reporting%20 currently% 20having%20depression].

Wohlwill, J. 1974. Human Adaptation to Levels of Environmental Stimulation. *Human Ecology* 2: 127–147.

Worster, D. 1994. *The Wealth of Nature: Environmental History and The Ecological Imagination*. Oxford: Oxford University Press.

Wuntu, C. N. 2014. James Fenimore Cooper and the Idea of Environmental Conservation in the Leatherstocking Tales (1823–1841). *Rubikon: Journal of Transnational American Studies* 1 (2): 25–38.

Wyckoff, W. and L. Dilsaver. 1995. *The Mountainous West: Explorations in Historical Geography*. Lincoln: University of Nebraska Press.

Yano, K. and K. Oishi. 2018. The Relationships Among Daily Exercise, Sensory- Processing Sensitivity, and Depressive Tendency in Japanese University Students. *Personality and Individual Differences* 127: 49–53.

Young, T. 2017. *Heading Out: A History of American Camping*. Ithaca: Cornell University Press.

Young, T. 2018. Frederick Law Olmsted's Abandoned San Francisco Park Plan. In *The American Environment Revisited*, edited by G. L. Buckley and Y. Youngs, 145–160. Lanham: Rowman & Littlefield.

Zeller, T. 2022. *Consuming Landscapes: What We See When We Drive and Why it Matters*. Baltimore: Johns Hopkins University Press.

Zierer, C. 1952. Tourism and Recreation in the West. *Geographical Review* 42 (3): 462–481.

Zimmerman, H. 2021. Predating the ADA, This Park County Camp is a Prime Example of Accessibility in Nature. *KUNC* 6 August. [https://www.kunc.org/news/2021-08-06 /predating-the-ada-this-park-county-camp-is-a-prime-example-of-accessibility-in -nature].

Index

About the Author

Jeffrey S. Smith is a cultural geographer whose work examines the relationships among place, landscape, and human experience. He earned his Ph.D. from Arizona State University, specializing in humanistic geography. His research focuses on sense of place, place attachment, restorative places, therapeutic landscapes, and the historical forces that have shaped Americans' engagement with the built environment.

Smith's teaching and fieldwork reflect this interdisciplinary approach. He regularly leads students into diverse landscapes of the American West (from the High Plains and the upper Rio Grande to the Colorado Plateau) using experiential learning to illuminate the connections between environment, culture, and identity. His upper-level courses emphasize place-based inquiry, the interpretation of cultural landscapes, and the value of field immersion in understanding geographic processes and meanings.

Across his scholarship and teaching, Smith brings together historical analysis, field observation, and theoretical perspectives from geography, history, and the social sciences to better understand how environments influence well-being and how people, in turn, shape the places they depend on.

www.ingramcontent.com/pod-product-compliance
Lightning Source LLC
LaVergne TN
LVHW091138140926
847902LV00025B/326

* 9 7 8 1 4 2 1 4 5 6 0 1 0 *